(The Many Health Benefits

Of Grapefruit Seed Extract (GSE))

(Why I wouldn't be without it & why this multipurpose

nutritional should be in *your* medicine cabinet)

(Michelle Oaks)

(The Many Health Benefits of Grapefruit Seed Extract (GSE))

Copyright © 2014 by (Michelle Oaks)

Photographer: Josh Oaks

ISBN-13: 978-1495249464

Printed in USA

'If I had only known the role that writing was going to play in my life, I would have paid better attention in English.'- Author Michelle Oaks

In memory of my mom, Carol Clark, 'the world is a much darker place without your light shining to diminish the darkness. We miss you more than words can say. We love you mom (Gma)'.

I want to thank Josh Oaks for his help with the photos for this book and for giving me reason to smile through all the tough times behind us & all the great times ahead.

We want to thank Mike (Michele) & Tom Hile for everything. You have no idea how much we appreciate you and everything you have done. Having you in our life has been a true blessing ☺

I want to thank Inga-Lil Sandstrom for being such a wonderful friend and sister of my heart. You are always there with a kind word. We appreciate you so much ☺

A thank you also goes out to Dana Burns & Tina Marie Howser and all of my other fans on my author page http://facebook.com/authormichelleoaks thank you for your support. It is greatly appreciated.

If you would like the opportunity to see your name in my next book please go over and like my page. Leaving comments gets you extra chances at having your name picked to be listed.

The Many Health Benefits of Grapefruit Seed Extract (GSE)

This book is for educational purposes to help you in conjunction with conventional treatment. It could also come in handy in the case of a national disaster, such as a SHTF scenario where you are on your own and this information could save the life of you and your family.

You can keep updated on Michelle Oaks's work here:

http://facebook.com/authormichelleoaks
http://oaksblogs.com/michelleoaks
http://twitter.com/michelleoaks3

Table of Contents

8

The Many Health Benefits of Grapefruit Seed Extract (GSE)

The grapefruit has long been used by dieters trying to lose weight but there is something that you may not know. Grapefruit contains something so powerful, so *amazing* that you will probably be surprised that such wonders can happen from the small seeds that the grapefruit contains.

Grapefruit seed extract has been confirmed to be 10 times more successful at killing household germs than Chlorine Bleach is. Imagine having that all of that power killing nasty germs and working to keep your family healthy.

This guide will show you how grapefruit seed extract is being used by many people worldwide to keep not only their families healthy but their pets as well. It can also be used for cleaning. And GSE is very economical.

Grapefruit seed extract is a multipurpose nutritional that should be in every home. Whether you believe in natural remedies, or just want to hedge your bets by having something on hand that you can use in an emergency, this is *it*.

I have an important question for you.

What would you do if you were out in the middle of nowhere, or in a SHTF scenario, and a loved one came down with an infection or parasites?

Simply having this little bottle in your medicine cabinet or in your camping gear could be a lifesaver.

Read this guide to find out the many uses of grapefruit seed extract.

As always, you should talk with your doctor before you take any herb, or natural remedy, as it may counteract with some medications.

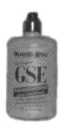

GSE Introduction

Before I begin I would like to say that there are some people out there that will pooh-pooh the use of grapefruit seed extract, and some might even take it further, but there are testimonials all over the internet of people who have used grapefruit seed extract.

These people have had wonderful experiences with grapefruit seed extract and aren't shy about telling anyone, and everyone, about how great it works.

I am one of them

Several years ago I had never even heard of grapefruit seed extract, otherwise known as GSE, and now?

Well, now I wouldn't be   without it.

Toxicity of Grapefruit Seed Extract

To be honest, I have seen people saying that people shouldn't use GSE because it contains toxins.

I suppose there is a possibility that maybe some brands might contain toxins but I have been using grapefruit seed extract for at least 7 years now without any issues. And truthfully when I think about how word is spreading about how great GSE works I could see that the big pharmaceutical companies could be concerned about losing their profits.

For that matter, I could see that they might be tempted to cause people to fear using grapefruit seed extract. The more people that heal themselves using natural remedies such as grapefruit seed extract the less money that the pharmaceutical companies will make.

I can't say that this is what is going on but in my opinion it could definitely be a possibility.

Anyway, I have not been what you would call 'loyal' to any certain brand as I always get whatever brand GSE I can get the easiest and the cheapest. Yet I have been happy with how well the GSE has worked each and every time that I have used it. So I really don't feel that, if you stick with the more reputable brands of grapefruit seed extract that, contamination should be a big concern.

I have read that the GSE brand Citricidal, had an Oral Toxicity Study done by North-view Pacific Labs. You can research this, the Report Number is X5E015G and it is dated 7/6/95.

The results of this study found that Citricidal is considered to be non-toxic by oral ingestion with an LD50 of over 5000 mg/kg of live body weight.

What that means is this:

A 200 pound person would need to drink close to 1 pound of pure Citricidal liquid every day for a whole two weeks, before there would even be the chance of a 50% risk of a fatal poisoning.

Now, since there are close to 20,000 drops in one pound of Citricidal liquid and the recommended adult dose is 5-10 drops at a time so you can see where you would have to drink a huge amount of grapefruit seed extract for it to be considered a toxicity threat.

The Extraordinary Cost per Dose of GSE

One more thing that I would like to mention in these financially difficult times is that grapefruit seed extract is very easy on the pocket. The average dose is approximately 5-10 drops. The last bottle of grapefruit seed extract that I bought was four ounces. The label states that a dose is 10 drops and that there are 400 doses in the bottle. This bottle cost me less than $15.00 and the shipping was free.

That comes out to less than 4 cents per *dose*!

That is extremely cheap for something that works so well against so many pathogens, is non-toxic, can be used for pets and even cleaning too!

My Experiences with Grapefruit Seed Extract

I, myself, have used the recommended dosage and I have used a much higher dosage. Now, even the higher dosage was still well below an amount that would come anywhere near being a 'toxic dose' but it was still on the high end of 'average' and yet I have had no problems.

Matter-of-fact, I have never had any bad reactions to the grapefruit seed extract *ever*.

Some people have stated that a higher dose upset their stomach but I have never had that happen even when I was putting 11 drops of liquid GSE into my 20 ounce bottle of juice, tea, pop, etc. This is despite my refilling that bottle probably 5-10 times or so a day, at this same strength of grapefruit seed extract, when my infection was at its worst.

I am not necessarily recommending this much GSE for just anyone but it was what I felt that I needed to do at the time because of the severity of the infection.

Yet despite using relatively large doses' and my using GSE for extended periods of time, I have only had good results. I have even had it improve other conditions besides what I was taking it for at the time.

Pre-GSE

I'll go back a bit so you can better understand why I even tried using grapefruit seed extract.

Since I was in my teens I have had trouble with ear/sinus infections. I have had ear infections multiple times a year which have always required me to be on antibiotics and quite often have been so bad that I am in terrible pain. Sometimes it has been to the point that I could barely eat, drink or even talk until the antibiotic started to take effect and the swelling went down some.

And I always seem to have sinus trouble whenever the weather changes back and forth from warm to cold to warm and then sometimes back to cold again. This means that pretty much every spring and every autumn I would get a sinus problem that would then go into a cold or a sinus infection.

Now I am sure that most of you are aware that going to the doctor and filling your prescriptions can be very expensive. And even though it was cheaper years ago than what it is now, it was still expensive at the time.

And nowadays we are all aware of the fact that antibiotics, and the misuse of them, are creating what are called super-bugs. So many of us are realizing how important it is not to use antibiotics unless they are *really* necessary.

Back then no one knew anything about that. Antibiotics were considered the miracle cure.

Now we realize that there could be a price to pay for all of that overuse of antibiotics.

With all of that in mind, when I heard about how wonderful grapefruit seed extract is, I decided to give it a try.

I have never, not even once, regretted that decision.

My Experience with GSE

Well, years ago when I discovered grapefruit seed extract, I had no idea the impact that it would have on my life.

As I started to say…before discovering GSE I used to get sinus infections every spring and autumn as well as any time in between.

As a result of this I have taken more rounds of antibiotics in my life than I care to even think about.

The last time I went to the doctor was years ago. The doctor wasn't even sure what was wrong but prescribed an expensive antibiotic because it was obvious I had a bad infection. Though, she couldn't tell if it was ear/sinus or an abscessed tooth or if the pain and swelling were the result of a combination of all three at work.

The nice thing about using grapefruit seed extract in a case like this is you don't even need to know exactly *where* the infection source is nor do you even need to know exactly *what* the source is-bacterial, fungal, viral, etc. GSE works for all of them and it works really well.

So anyway, I got the expensive antibiotics, went home and proceeded to take them as prescribed. They helped some but when they were gone I still had the infection and my medical insurance had run out.

I had been using natural healing methods for years and had only gone to the doctor because at that time a friend convinced me that I should go to the doctor before my health insurance was gone.

Having gone to the doctor I had stopped all natural healing methods so there would be no opportunity for an adverse reaction between the two 'medicines'.

Up until I decided to write this book I had always looked back on that incident with regret that I had gone to the doctor and stopped my natural healing remedies while using conventional antibiotics.

After all, the antibiotics didn't get rid of the infection so I felt that I would have been further ahead to have continued the natural remedies as I had for years before with great success.

Now though I look back at that as my own personal experiment pitting natural remedies against conventional therapy and found that *in my experience* that the natural remedy won.

After finishing my round of antibiotics and still having the infection active I started on grapefruit seed extract and some vitamin C thrown in for good measure. It wasn't long and I felt so much better and soon the infection was completely gone.

A Recent Experience of Mine

I myself have been taking grapefruit seed extract on a long term basis, with some small breaks in between, and have not noticed any ill effects. Frankly it's not hard to use Grapefruit seed extract frequently with all of the illnesses that it is good for.

Recently I had a very bad infection which resulted in swelling of my face and glands, terrible pain to the point of hardly being able to stand it even when I would use a couple of Extra Strength Acetaminophen every 4-6 hours along with reflexology for pain.

Now, I don't use acetaminophen very often but this pain was so bad that I was desperate for some relief.

Anyway, not seeing any relief to speak of after using the acetaminophen, reflexology and a topical analgesic I happened to remember reading that grapefruit seed extract is good for pain.

I was already using grapefruit seed extract for the infection, and it was helping, but I was not using a very high concentration of it. I used a few drops about three times a day.

Then I happened to remember reading about a drunken agricultural worker in Peru accidentally drank four fluid ounces of grapefruit seed extract because of someone playing a prank on him.

It seems that the only affect that the GSE had on him was to clear out all of the numerous parasites that he had in his body. It is said that even at that concentration that this man did not have any ill effects.

Thinking on that I realized that I should safely be able to increase my dosage, to see if it would actually help for the pain, without worry about harmful effects.

Well, it seemed to me that my infection was so bad that it was creating a horrible pressure underneath my teeth. So any time my teeth bumped against each other- no matter how careful I was or how gently it would happen- it sent excruciating pain shooting through me.

Now at one point the swelling was so bad that the pressure on the nerves actually cut of the pain signals and, despite the terrible swelling, I had no pain. Of course once the swelling started to come down I was again in pain.

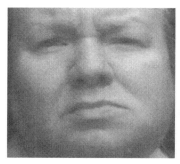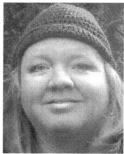

Me with my swollen face - how my face usually looks

The picture of my face swollen was after the swelling had come down enough that I was in excruciating pain as you can tell by my forehead. My mouth area was so swollen that my lip was puffed up, my left eye was nearly swollen shut and misery is clearly written on my face.

Anyway, since I had also read that tests have shown grapefruit seed extract to be very nontoxic, I decided to try up my intake of GSE in order to kill the infection and help for the pain.

In fact, I have read that research has indicated that a person weighing 180lbs would need to consume around 5.5 pints of a 50% solution of GSE in order for them to become severely poisoned.

That's a LOT of GSE.

Before I finish my story I want to talk about brands of GSE for just a minute as it is germane to the story and I believe that many will be wondering about if it makes a difference or not.

Does Brand Really Matter?

I don't believe so. I feel that if you stick with some of the better known brands then you should be ok and the grapefruit seed extract should work well.

I will say that I recently switched from the brand that I had just run out of to another one due to a huge difference in cost. Since I have tried several brands and they all seem to work very well I wasn't concerned about switching brands. But I *did* notice a difference between them.

It wasn't really a matter of a difference in how well each brand worked.

It was more a matter of taste.

Here is what happened…

When I upped my intake of GSE to kill the infection and to help with the pain I started putting 11 drops of grapefruit seed extract in my 20 fluid ounce bottle that I like to use to mix my 'GSE drink' in and carry with me so that I don't have to worry about it spilling and I always have some of my GSE ready to drink (when I am sick like this at least).

Since the toxic dose for GSE is so high, and the infection was so bad, I kept putting 11 drops in every time that I refilled my drinking bottle throughout the day. Which as it happened was quite a few times.

To my amazement it did help for the pain quite quickly and in a few days I was feeling so much better and the swelling was down.

But, like with any medicine you need to continue taking it for a while even after you feel better just to be sure that all the infection is gone and the medicine has completed its job.

Well, I felt so much better that I quit taking the grapefruit seed extract and started overdoing things and it wasn't long and I relapsed.

Well, my grapefruit seed extract was nearly gone so we had to make an emergency run to a town approximately 45 miles away to get a new bottle of GSE as no one seems to carry it anywhere closer to us than that.

***Note to self-try to keep a spare bottle of GSE on hand for emergencies like this.

***Note to you- you might want to learn from my mistake. ☺

Anyway, luckily they had a bottle.

So this time, when I had my bottle of grapefruit seed extract about half gone, I decided that I should get another bottle soon so that I would not run out.

I ordered a 4 ounce bottle online which is four times as big as the bottles that I have been buying. It was a different brand but I had used that brand before.

Little did I realize the difference in the two bottles of GSE. The first time that I used any of the grapefruit seed extract out of the new bottle I added the 11 drops. Mixed it well and took a drink.

Boy was it bitter!

I didn't realize what a difference in taste that there could be between brands like that.

BUT, I cut my dose down to 2-4 drops at a time and it wasn't nearly as bitter tasting. Of course it then meant I had to drink more to get the same amount of grapefruit seed extract into me. After a while though I became more used to the taste and have begun adding more drops again.

Heel Spurs

When I was little I noticed that I had a whole bunch of white 'balls' in the heel of my foot. No one else that I knew had these. As a little girl I thought that it was really something that I had these and no one else did.

As I grew I noticed that I always had them. They never seemed to get larger or increase in number and they never went away.

At some point I found out that they were called 'heel spurs' and as a teenager I found out that from older people that they weren't so great after all.

Now, I haven't really had any issues with them. Sometimes my feet hurt but since I am on them a lot I think it's more from that rather than from the heel spurs. And the pain doesn't originate in the heel so my heel spurs were never a problem for me.

But recently I was thinking about putting grapefruit seed extract on them to see if it would make them go away as I had heard of others using GSE for their heel spurs.

I was going to be a 'guinea pig', so to speak, as much for curiosity sake as to better inform you.

But, when I checked my heel spurs…..

They Were GONE!

After having had them all of my life, and not having done anything to get rid of them, I cannot find a single one. I had so many of them that I cannot believe that they are completely gone but they are.

I don't have a before pic- for which I am kicking myself. But, since I had made no effort to get rid of them I had no idea that my taking the GSE for infections and other issues would get rid of my heel spurs.

So, while I can include a picture that will show you that I don't have them any more I cannot show you a before picture as I don't go around taking pictures of my feet for no reason ☺ lol.

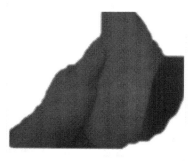

Get to Know More about Grapefruit Seed Extract

Grapefruit seed extract comes from the small seeds found within each grapefruit.

Grapefruit seed extract is also known as GSE. It is created by processing the seeds, pulp and even the white membrane of the grapefruit.

The manufacturing process converts the polyphenolics found in grapefruit into a very powerful substance that has been verified to be extremely successful in a wide range of uses.

GSE has been found to be effective even at very low concentrations so a little can go a long way.

GSE has become well known for its amazing benefits and is now frequently being added to a large variety of nutritional supplements and other household items.

GSE is a multipurpose nutritional that really should be in pretty much everyone's medicine cabinet.

A four ounce bottle of grapefruit seed extract contains something like 4000 drops of this powerful natural antibiotic and multipurpose nutritional.

As I stated above, grapefruit seed extract is a multipurpose nutritional. In this book I am going to tell you about the ways that grapefruit seed extract are being used not only for humans but for animals too.

Grapefruit Seed Extract GSE contains bio-flavonoids such as quercetin and others that are very effective against infections.

Infections such as:

Bacteria
Fungi
Protozoa
Viruses

Grapefruit seed extract is known to be a powerful anti-oxidant rich in bio-flavonoids and polyphenolic compounds. They also are loaded with vitamins A and vitamin C which are known to strengthen our immune system.

GSE is around 50,000 on the ORAC scale which details food's antioxidant capacity. That shows us that grapefruit seed extract is a powerful antioxidant.

Grapefruit seed extract is also known for being highly alkaline which works to alkalinize your body if it is too acidic. This creates a hostile environment for harmful microorganisms such as bacteria and fungi.

Grapefruit seed extract does wonderful things for humans and pets. It is tremendously powerful while also being safe and effective.

You may be wondering what kind of side effects you can expect, especially if you use it regularly?

Well the good news is that, as far as studies have shown thus far, there aren't any known side effects using GSE. Studies have found that GSE does not have any bad effects even with continuing treatment.

GSE can be taken for 1-3 months or even longer if necessary without harmful side effects

Though some people like to take a short break from taking GSE every few weeks when taking it on a long term basis it is not a necessity.

Numerous studies have followed people who have been taking GSE for a year or more. These studies have found no conclusive evidence proving that there are any detrimental side effects to using grapefruit seed extract.

***A word of caution though for anyone who is taking medications as: they should use grapefruit seed extract with caution. There is a possibility that it could interact with certain medications and possibly create unwanted results. It would be a good idea to check with doctor or nutritionist before using grapefruit seed extract.

***Pregnant women and breastfeeding mothers should also talk with their doctor before taking grapefruit seed extract.

***You should also avoid using GSE when you are taking blood pressure medication.

Adverse Effects

If you consult your doctor and be sure to take the correct dose then you shouldn't need to worry about detrimental side effects. A lot of laboratories have tested GSE since as far back as 1974. To date there haven't been any reported negative side effects from using grapefruit seed extract.

Since grapefruit seed extract is all-natural there are very few negative side effects.

Currently, there has been no irrefutable evidence showing that GSE interacts with any other drug.

Studies have shown that drug interactions that are caused by drinking fresh grape fruit juice do not exist with grape fruit seed extract. GSE does not contain the same ingredients that are found in grape fruit juice that hinder some medications.

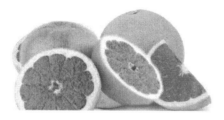

Citrus Allergies

Now, if you are allergic to citrus then I would say that grapefruit seed extract is probably not for you. But if you were allergic to citrus then chances are you never would have been interested in this book in the first place.

Researchers estimate that only 3 to 5% of the people are allergic to citrus fruits.

If you happen to be allergic then you may possibly have a reaction to grape fruit seed extract. But, from my understanding, not everyone that is allergic to citrus has an adverse reaction to GSE.

If you are allergic to citrus fruits but you would like to still give GSE an attempt then you should talk with your health care provider and if you both decide for you to try GSE then you should take care to start with a very small dose.

Legally I cannot recommend for someone who is allergic to citrus to use GSE but I can say what I would say to you if you were a friend who had gotten the go ahead from their doctor.

First of all, from my understanding, it seems that the probability of having an adverse reaction to grapefruit seed extract is small. Since the benefits are so great, if you feel that the benefits outweigh the risk, then I would consider trying GSE.

But, it is a personal decision that only you can make and should only be done after your doctor has approved it.

You should also keep in mind the following points first:

How allergic are you?

Weigh the pros and cons of trying GSE

How bad is the infection or other health issue?

Do you have someone there that could help you if you did have a reaction?

What time of day is it? If I were to try it I would be sure to do so early in the morning so that if you were to have a reaction you would have a better chance of getting good medical care.

I would also be sure to have a bottle of vitamin C on hand as it is a natural antihistamine.

Then after weighing all of this and deciding to go ahead and try grape fruit seed extract I would do these two things to be on the safe side.

First of all, I would perform a patch test:

In a clean small glass or ceramic bowl mix 1 drop of GSE with either 1 or 2 drops of water. Then dip a cotton swab in this solution and swab it on a small area on your wrist/arm area. Cover this with a band-aid and wait.

Check it is 24 hours and again in 48 hours. If you have no reaction to this application of GSE, then move on to trying a very dilute dose internally as mentioned below.

If you have any reaction then quickly wash the area and monitor how you feel and how it looks for the next few days. If anything happens that you question, or concerns you, then you should have a professional look at you as soon as possible.

If all goes well with the patch test then....

Secondly I would try an extremely low dose of grapefruit seed extract if I still want to try it,

When I say low dose I am talking about putting 1 drop in a cup of water, mix well, and then just try a teaspoon or less. Wait 1-2 hours or so and then if you have no reaction you might try another spoonful or so.

Then I would wait until the next day to try again only this time I would try a little more and then you could work your way up on your dosage if there are no problems.

***Never take GSE full-strength- Always be sure to dilute GSE with water or juice.

***If you get GSE into your eyes you should flush them out immediately with plenty of warm water for at least 15 minutes.

Benefits of Grapefruit Seed Extract

Grapefruit has long been known to have many health benefits.

Grapefruit seed extract is made from the seeds and the pulp.

Grapefruit seed extract is a very acidic liquid. Though GSE is acidic, it actually creates an alkaline environment in the body when taking it.

GSE contains bio-flavonoids, as well as vitamin C and E. These well known antioxidants help our body to fight against free radicals and they help to sustain the correct metabolism in our body.

GSE contains what are known as polyphenolic compounds.

These include:

Quercitin

Helperidin

Naringin

Rutinoside

Grapefruit seed extract has long been used by many alternative medicine practitioners because of its healing ability. The wonderful healing properties in GSE are, in part, due to the polyphenolic compounds it contains. They are considered to be anti-carcinogenic, anti-inflammatory, and antioxidant.

GSE is also a great natural antibiotic as it helps the body to fight all sorts of bacterial, fungal and viral infections.

Grapefruit seed extract is very effective for cleaning the garbage out of your body. It also balances out the systems in your body.

Because of grapefruit seed extracts wonderful therapeutic importance it can benefit your health in many ways. It is wonderful to have on hand to fight many diseases.

And grapefruit seed extract, unlike conventional antibiotics, does not create drug resistant bacteria.

So far there is no evidence that pathogenic microorganisms have ever built up a resistance to the active ingredient found in grapefruit seed extract.

Because grapefruit seed extract disrupts the cytoplasmic membrane of organisms it is believed that it is impossible for bacteria to build up any sort of resistance to it.

Grapefruit seed extract can be used for humans and pets such as:

Birds

Cats

Dogs

Fish

Reptiles & more

Pretty much any, and all, living creatures have benefited from using grapefruit seed extract.

Grapefruit seed extract is considered to be a multipurpose product because it can be used for numerous applications:

Basic GSE Wash

This basic grapefruit seed extract wash can be kept, ready to use, in a spray bottle for cleaning, wound care and numerous uses around your home and yard.

Use a:

Clean16 oz spray bottle

Add 30-40 drops of grapefruit seed extract

Then fill the bottle with water

Shake to mix well

Be sure to shake well before each use as the grapefruit seed extract tends to settle to the bottom after sitting for a while.

Gardening Uses

Bug spray

Plant spray

Remove fungus and molds on plants, tools, etc.

Tool cleaner

Household Uses

Counter tops- 30-60 drops of GSE in a 32 oz. pump sprayer bottle filled with water. Mix well and use this on pretty much every surface around your home.

Cutting boards- apply 10-20 drops to cutting board and work into the board with a dish cloth. Leave it on for at least 30 minutes and then rinse with water.

Laundry cleaner

Add GSE to your final rinse to kill pathogens.

Produce wash

Use GSE to kill bacteria, parasites, etc. on your fruits and vegetables. This comes in handy with all of the e-coli scares in recent years. This also helps to remove pesticides, wax, etc.

Human Health

Internal and external conditions

Infections

GSE works wonderfully well on pretty much any type of infection as it is effective against so many different bacteria, fungus, viruses, parasites, etc.

Viruses

You hear how 'antibiotics don't work against viruses' and how you just have to drink plenty of fluids and get a lot of bed rest. Well grapefruit seed extract does work against viruses so now you don't have to just lie down and take it any more. You can fight back by using GSE,

You can use it as a preventative or after you have become exposed. If you catch it quick enough you might not even become ill or you might just feel a little 'under the weather' for a couple of days.

Even if you are too late and are already sick, by taking GSE you can lessen the severity of the symptoms and shorten the duration of your illness.

And many other conditions listed in full elsewhere in this book.

Pet Health

Internal and external conditions

Infections-

Give animal the maintenance dose listed for its size in the dosage chart on page 169.
Give this dosage 3-5 times daily until better. Then it is a good idea to give the maintenance dose at least once per day for a few days after that.

Skin conditions-

Thoroughly mix 30 to 40 drops of GSE liquid extract in a quart of water. You can then spray this on the infected area.

OR you can mix the grapefruit seed extract into their shampoo. Wet skin, or fur, soap up and then leave this on their skin or fur for a few minutes. Rinse well.

Mange-

You will need to thoroughly mix 30 to 40 drops of GSE liquid extract in a quart of water. You can then spray this on the infected area several times a day until the mange is gone.

It would be a good idea to continue to spray the area once or twice a day for several days even after the mange seems to be gone just to help prevent re-infestation of the fungus.

Fleas

You will need to shampoo your pet's fur thoroughly with a mix of 5-10 drops of grapefruit seed extract mixed into a tablespoon of your usual shampoo. Then work it into a good lather into the wet hair of your pet. Make sure not to get this into the animals' eyes,

Once lathered up then leave it on for several minutes and then rinse it well.

Repeat this procedure in 3 days and continue to do so often throughout the flea season.

For really stubborn cases you can add a few drops of grapefruit seed extract to a spoonful of olive oil & then rub this solution in to the animals' fur a couple of times each day during flea infestations.

***Do *not* allow them to lick this concentrated mixture as it could irritate their tongue.

Travel Uses

Diarrhea   Dysentery

Food borne illnesses   Water borne illnesses

It would be a good idea, not just for these issues, but just the fact that you are away from home to have a bottle of grapefruit seed extract on hand as you never know when you might need it.

It would be a terrible thing for you to be on a business trip, or a vacation, and have an illness ruin it or send you home early.

List of the Health Benefits of Grapefruit Seed Extract

Items highlighted in yellow were found listed in numerous sources but more information was not found.

***NOTE- I have only had experience with liquid grapefruit seed extract. So, I cannot say how well the capsules and tablets work.

With that said, I know that some of you won't like the taste (bitterness) of some brands of liquid GSE so you probably won't use GSE unless it would be in pill form.

So, I came across this information and thought that it might come in handy for some of you.

10 - 15 drops = 1 - 2 capsules/tablets

Aids-HIV positive

I was reading about how a growing number of HIV positive people are finding relief in using GSE to boost their immune system in fighting bacteria, fungus, viruses and parasites.

Now, as their immune systems are already taxed enough it is very important that these people start with a very dilute solution and build up slowly.

Doing this lessens the burden that will be put on their weakened immune system by not creating a strong Herxheimer Reaction.

You need to build up your immune system starting with a low dose and gradually build up the amount of grapefruit seed extract.

So, for HIV positive people you might want to start with 1 drop of GSE each day until you are comfortable with how you are feeling and then slowly increase your dose.

If 1 drop of grapefruit seed extract seems to create a strong detoxifying effect then you may want to cut back and increase your dose more slowly. This can be done by mixing 1 drop of GSE into a cup of water, juice, tea, etc. Then only drink a portion of that to get a half of a drop or a quarter of a drop to start.

A strong detoxifying effect is recognized by these symptoms:

Diarrhea

Fever (with or without chills)

Flushing

Headaches

Heavy perspiration and night sweats

Itching

Malaise

Nausea and vomiting

Pain in joints and bones

Rashes or skin lesions

Sore muscles

***Be sure to check with your doctor before starting to use grapefruit seed extract, or anything else, that may interfere with any conventional protocol that your doctor has you on.

Alkalizing:

GSE is wonderful for alkalizing the body. And as you may have heard a lot of health benefits can be had by keeping your body at the proper ph balance. Grapefruit seed extract is believed to be one of the most alkaline forming foods there is.

GSE is the most alkalizing of all the fruits. Raising the pH of your body so that it is an alkaline state, rather than acidic, is thought to be one of the most important health regeneration benefits to be had.

It has been found that disease cannot survive in an alkaline environment. Researchers claim that cancerous cells die in an alkaline environment.

8.0 is the PH level at which cancerous cells die.

The pH of a healthy person is approximately 7.5.

Disease causing microforms cannot survive in an alkaline environment because an alkaline environment is highly oxygenated.

Disease causing microforms such as:

Bacteria

Fungi

Parasites

Viruses

Many conditions and diseases are caused by an acid environment so restoring the proper pH can alleviate these conditions and diseases.

Lots of the foods that we eat on a regular basis are actually acid forming foods. Foods such as meats, sugary foods and most grains cause the environment within our body to become acidic.

Yet many acidic foods actually have an alkaline effect on the body. GSE has a pH of 2.0 and yet it has an extremely alkalizing effect on our body. This can bring about some wonderful health benefits.

Allergies

Using a preventative dose of 1-4 drops of grapefruit seed extract mixed in a cupful of water 2-3 times a day can help your body when dealing with allergies.

You may want to start this dosage ahead of known allergy seasons for you.

Antibiotic

When infection is present it is usually necessary to use antibiotics to kill the infection before it spreads. But, nowadays we are being told about super-germs that are the result of overuse of antibiotics. And we are warned that it this trend continues we may not have many choices when it comes to infections.

The good news is that with grapefruit seed extract the bacteria, parasites and viruses do not seem to become immune to the GSE as they do with many common modern antibiotics that are in use today

As a preventative & for good health

Since grapefruit seed extract kills bacteria, parasites, viruses, etc. It is good to use as a preventative measure. This is especially important for people in certain types of jobs.

If you are a person who cares for anyone for which getting sick could be a big concern, such as young children or the elderly, GSE should be your first line of   defense.

If you work in a doctors office and come into contact with sick people on a regular basis and yet you do not want to be bringing home all these germs to your family… GSE should be in your medicine cabinet.

If you cannot afford to miss time from work… you should have GSE on hand to use as a preventative and to be able to start dosing yourself at the first sign of an illness or when you *know* that you were just exposed to someone sick.

I have found that any time Josh or I are starting to feel the first signs of coming down with something, or we know that we were just exposed to someone who is sick; or that we are really busy, not getting enough sleep, exposed to cold damp weather- in other words our immune system is being stressed and we are not getting the sleep we need to recharge it- then we simply have a drop or two of grapefruit seed extract once or twice a day for a couple of days and we seem to avoid getting sick.

You can also use it to sanitize your hands, door knobs and other surfaces to kill germs and halt the spread of the illness.

Athlete's foot

Athlete's foot is called tinea pedi , or ringworm of the foot. It is caused by a fungus and is a form of ringworm.

The fungus that causes athlete's foot is Trichophyton. It is commonly found on floors, and in clothing. Even so, only about 0.75% of people who walk barefoot regularly even get it.

Conditions have to be   right for it to develop:

Warm

Moist

Irritated

Athlete's foot is recognized by the following symptoms:

Burning

Dry flaky skin

Itching

Red scaly skin

Stinging

In more advanced cases it can cause:

Cracks in the skin

Crusting blisters

Oozing

Swelling

And severe cases can have raw, open cracks that can be prone to infection.

In South America grapefruit seed extract is being used in public swimming pools instead of using chlorine because GSE

Does not cause skin irritation

Does not evaporate in warmer temperature

Has no harmful vapor

Is not decomposed by UV rays

Leaves no toxic residue

GSE iIs active against a range of fungi-including athletes' foot which typically flourishes in the environment of a swimming pool.

Commercial preparations for athlete's foot that contain grape fruit seed extract have been found to be quite helpful.

Bad Breath

Bad Breath is usually caused by bacteria running rampant inside the mouth. Tooth decay or putrefaction in the lower digestive tract can also cause bad breath otherwise known as halitosis. Grapefruit seed extract is particularly effective and a long lasting breath freshener.

Benign Tumors, Cysts, Lymphomas, Polyps, and Wens

You are supposed to be able to use grapefruit seed extract to shrink Benign Tumors, Cysts, Lymphomas, Polyps, and Wens. Some people state that they applied a drop directly to the abnormality but others stated that they mixed the GSE with carrier oil such as coconut oil or olive oil.

Bladder Infections, Chronic Urethritis and Interstitial Cystitis

This type of infection is commonly recognized by cloudy urine and a bad odor. The pain usually goes away while urinating but then it quickly returns.

Cranberry juice is widely recommended as a home remedy. You should also drink plenty of water to flush the bacteria out. But you can also use GSE to kill the bacteria.

Broad Spectrum Antibiotic

What seems to be the most common reason for people taking grapefruit seed extract is its amazing ability to work both externally and internally against a large variety of infections that are caused by bacteria, funguses parasites and viruses.

According to numerous published sources, grapefruit seed extract is considered to be useful against over 800 different bacterial and viral strains, a large number of single-cell and multi-celled parasites, as well as 100 different strains of fungus.

GSE is a preventative as it can be taken for long periods of time without any toxic side effects. There have been people that have reported taking grapefruit seed extract every day for several years, simply as a preventative, without any detrimental side effects.

I, myself, have personally taken GSE pretty much every day now for two years. I have not had any bad reactions, or detrimental side effects, and have only noticed positive effects.

Candida infection

1st week: 1 drop taken twice a day in a cup of water
2nd week: 3 drops taken twice a day in a cup of water.
3rd week: 5-7 drops taken three times a day in a cup of water.

Drink plenty of water to help to flush the bacteria, and the toxins from the dying bacteria, out.

Candida Yeast

Mix 1-3 drops in a cup of water. Douche one time each day for 7-9 days.

Be sure to always dilute the GSE.

Candida, Vaginal Rinse and Yeast Infections

Mix 1-3 drops of GSE in 1 cup warm water to douche with. Use this solution one time each day for a week or as otherwise instructed to do by your doctor.

Make sure that you always dilute the grapefruit seed extract in warm water before using.

Chicken pox

Thoroughly mix 3 drops of GSE with a tablespoon of olive oil.
Apply this to the affected areas of the skin.
Alternatively you can mix 3-6 drops of GSE into 8 ounces
of water and spray this solution onto the affected area when
needed.
In addition it is a good idea to use GSE internally- see Antibiotic
dosage in Human Uses- General Use

Colds and Flu:

Using grapefruit seed extract at the first sign of a cold or flu could
stop colds and the flu in its tracks. Even if you don't catch it quick
enough the GSE should lessen the symptoms while also decreasing
the duration of your illness. So, it's most definitely worth using
grapefruit seed extract.

Cold sores

Cold sores are caused by a virus and since grapefruit seed extract
kills viruses it works well for ridding the body of the cold sore
virus

Coughs, Hoarseness and Laryngitis

Mix 3-5 drops in 1 cup lukewarm water and then use this solution to gargle 3-5 times a day.

Also, ingesting a mixture of 2-3 drops of GSE several times a day will help to boost your immune system.

Crohn's disease

There are some experts that say that many people that are diagnosed with colitis or crohn's disease are actually infected with parasites. GSE is very effective against parasites so if these experts are correct then it would be possible that grapefruit seed extract would kill said parasites and in doing so take care of the symptoms known as crohn's disease.

Chronic Fatigue Syndrome

You need to build up your immune system starting with a low dose and gradually build up the amount of grapefruit seed extract until you are at the rcommended dosage for colds and flu which is:

3-5 drops in 1 cup water and take this 2-3 times a day

So, for chronic fatigue syndrome you might want to start with 1 drop of GSE each day until you are comfortable with how you are feeling.

You do not want to use too much GSE too quickly as you could have a bad detox reaction due to too much die off happening so quickly that your body is unable to cope with the sudden flood of toxins.

So it is especially important that you start small and build up to the recommended dose.

Chronic Inflammation

Chronic Inflammation is a symptom indicating that there is a weakening of the immune system which needs to be addressed.

Dental Caries/Tooth Decay

Dental caries is actually caused by the demineralization of the tooth enamel and the hard substance of the tooth. This is caused by the metabolic practice of plaque bacteria. Keeping teeth clean, using GSE to kill bacteria in your mouth and eating mineral rich foods can help to keep your teeth healthy and cavity-free.

Dental Rinse:

Using GSE diluted in water will kill damaging oral bacteria to help to keep your mouth healthy.

Diarrhea and Dysentery

Diarrhea and Dysentery are caused by bacterially contaminated food or water. Experts say that a lot of people that are diagnosed with either colitis or Crohn's disease might actually be infected with one of the following:

Amoebas   Fungi

Giardia lamblia   Parasites

Salmonella   Shigella

Grapefruit seed extract is extremely effective against these. Just be sure to start slow and to drink plenty of water because if you try to kill these off too quickly you can suffer from 'die-off' where your body has to deal with the toxins being released when these bacteria, fungus or parasites are killed.

Digestive disturbances

Many digestive issues come about due to pathogens which can be helped by the use of GSE.

Ear infections

Take 2-7 drops diluted in water several times a day orally.

You should also mix 1 to 5 drops of GSE in 1 oz vegetable glycerin or alcohol in a dropper bottle.

When needed just put 2 to 5 drops of mixture in affected ear as often as necessary.

***Do not use full strength in ears.

Ear Rinse

Thoroughly mix 1-3 drops of grapefruit seed extract with 1 ounce of vegetable glycerin   or alcohol.

Apply 1-2 drops of this solution in affected ears several times a day.

NEVER use full strength GSE in your ears

Earaches

Mix 1 to 5 drops of GSE in 1 oz vegetable glycerin or alcohol in a dropper bottle.

When needed just put 2 to 5 drops of mixture in affected ear as often as necessary.

***Do not use full strength in ears.

Economical

GSE is very efficient even at low concentrations, so a little goes a long way. Most uses will only need just a few drops per dose.

A 1 oz bottle usually contains approximately 600 drops so you can see that even a one ounce bottle would last for a while.

Epstein Barr Virus

. For Epstein Barr syndrome you should take 12 drops of grapefruit seed extract in water. Drink this solution 3 times every day.

External Skin Conditions

Many different types of external skin conditions, from both known and unknown causes, can be helped with grapefruit seed extract. This includes causes such as:

Bacteria

Fungal

Parasites

Viral

It is also effective to fight against fungal infections of the feet, nails and the skin.

Facial Cleanser for Oily Skin

Grapefruit seed extract is a good facial cleanser for oily skin and is quite good for fighting acne. You just need to apply 1-2 drops of GSE to your moistened fingertips and then you should gently massage your face, in a circular motion, for about a minute or so. Then you should rinse your face thoroughly with warm water.

Some people have reported a tingling sensation after using the GSE treatment. This is simply a sign that the grapefruit seed extract is working and deep cleaning your skin.

Flatulence (Gas)

Thoroughly mix 2- 5 drops of GSE in a cup of water and drink this solution 3 times a day.

Taking a pro-biotic would help to replenish beneficial bacteria in your digestive tract which could help to lessen these symptoms.

Food sensitivities

Fungal Infections

1st week: 1 drop taken twice a day in a cup of water
2nd week: 3 drops taken twice a day in a cup of water.
3rd week: 5-7 drops taken three times a day in a cup of water

Ulcers- Gastritis, Gastric and Duodenal

Helicobacter pylori is the bacteria now believed to be the underlying cause of as many as 90% of all peptic and duodenal ulcers.

If this bacteria is successfully treated, permanent relief is usually found.

Thoroughly mix 1- 5 drops of grapefruit seed extract in a cup of water. Drink 30 minutes before eating.

Do this 2 to 3 times a day until symptoms have disappeared. Then continue for an extra few days.

If your stomach is sensitive then you should start off with one drop in a cup of water. If that still bothers then you may try that strength of solution but only sip on it throughout the day so that you are getting a very dilute amount in any given time.

Then increase your dosage as needed until you get to the recommended dose.

***Note- since ulcers are very sensitive to acidic irritation care must be taken when using GSE. If the irritation persists then you should discontinue using the grapefruit seed extract as ulcers can be a very serious.

You should talk with your doctor about this issue.

Gastrointestinal Disorder

If the cause of your gastrointestinal disorder seems to be unknown then it is possible that you may be infected with:

Amoebas

Fungi

Giardia

Lamblia

Salmonella

Shigella

Or some other type of parasite that came from contaminated food, water, etc.

Gum disorders

Gum disorders are usually caused by the build up of bacteria which can be greatly reduced by the regular use of GSE.

Heel Spurs

Even though I talked about this earlier in the book I think for someone who is having issues with heel spurs then this story bears repeating. When I think about how GSE improved my heel spurs I am still amazed and feel that it could help others too.

Here's my story:

When I was little I noticed that I had a whole bunch of white 'balls' in the heel of my foot. No one else that I knew had these. As a little girl I thought that it was really something that I had these and no one else did.

As I grew I noticed that I always had them. They never seemed to get larger or increase in number and they never went away.

At some point I found out that they were called 'heel spurs' and as a teenager I found out that they weren't so great after all.

Now, I haven't really had any issues with them. Sometimes my feet hurt but since I am on them a lot I think it's more from that rather than from the heel spurs.

But recently I was thinking about trying potting grapefruit seed extract on them to see if it would make them go away as I had heard of others using GSE for their heel spurs.

I was going to be a 'guinea pig', so to speak, as much for curiosity sake as to better inform you.

But, when I checked my heel spurs…..

They Were GONE!

After having had them all of my life, and not having done anything to get rid of them, I cannot find a single one. I had so many of them that I cannot believe that they are completely gone but they are.

I don't have a before pic- for which I am kicking myself. But I can show you that I don't have them any more.

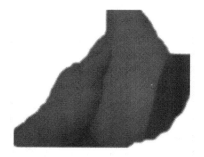

Herpes

Herpes is caused by a virus. Grapefruit seed extract works great against viruses.

A simple solution can be made to apply externally while also using the GSE internally.

Hypoallergenic:

GSE is considered to be pretty much non-allergenic. Dr. Allen Sachs says that only about 3-5% of people are allergic to citrus fruit. These people could therefore be more apt to be sensitive to GSE.

Anyone with an allergy to citrus should

1. **Get your doctors okay**
2. **Perform a patch test**
3. **Start with a very dilute solution as stated earlier in this book.**

Internal Cleansing

Feel like you need to clean house internally you can do an internal cleansing by adding 10 - 15 drops of grapefruit seed extract to a glass of juice and drink it. You do this three times a day.

Now if you need to work, or be able to leave your home for any reason you may want to schedule your cleanse for a time when leaving home for long periods of time will not be an issue.

Intestinal Amebiasis and giardiasis

These are parasites that can cause you to become quite ill. Using GSE against these seems to be quite effective for these parasites.

Pyorrhea

Pyorrhea is a gum disorder. Using grapefruit seed extract helps to keep your mouth healthy.

Ringworm

Ringworm is a fungal condition that can be found on humans and animals alike. A solution of GSE applied on a regular basis can kill the fungus and help the skin to heal.

Stimulates the immune system

GSE helps your immune system by greatly reducing the bacterial fungal or viral load while also stimulating your immune system.

Doctors and Veterinarians agree that GSE, taken in normal doses, is gentle to your system but it is not harmful to your beneficial bacteria.

Sore throat

Mix 1-7 drops of GSE in 4 ounces of water. Use this solution to gargle with several times a day.

Sinusitis

Mix 1-6 drops of GSE with 3/4 cup of tepid water.

See dosage section for further instructions

Toxic Shock Syndrome

If you use tampons you may worry about Toxic Shock Syndrome. TSS is a fairly rare but very dangerous disease.

As a protective measure you can douche with grapefruit seed extract. Mix a solution of 1 to 5 drops GSE in 1quart of warm water to use as a douche in order to kill rampant bacterial growth

Urinary tract infection

Urinary tract infections are caused by germs causing an infection.

You are prone to urinary tract infections if you...

Are a woman – women are more prone to UTI's because they have shorter urethras

Are pregnant

Do not drink enough water

Have diabetes

UTI symptoms include:

Belly feels tender

Feel like you have to urinate more often

Pain or burning sensation when urinating

Urine is cloudy or smells bad

Contact your doctor right away if you:

Are pregnant

Have pain on 1 side of back under ribs

Have diabetes, kidney disease or a compromised immune system

Or if you have:

Fever

Chills

Nausea

Vomiting

Or are over 65 years old

Cranberry juice is widely recommended as a home remedy. You should also drink plenty of water to flush the bacteria out. But you can also use GSE to kill the bacteria.

Weight loss

Eating grapefruit and drinking grapefruit juice has long been touted to be a weight loss remedy.

Since using GSE on a regular basis I have noticed that I don't seem to gain weight as easy and have actually lost weight without even going on a diet.

I cannot guarantee that you will lose weight just by using GSE but it seems to be helping me and in my research I came across others who mentioned about it helping them to lose weight.

It may depend on how much you take. But, if you have health issues and use the grapefruit seed extract for them you might find losing weight to be a nice little side benefit. ☺

Wound Healing:

GSE is excellent for healing wounds, and has been reported to even be good for healing scar tissue related to many wounds. Some have reported that GSE even works on big ugly scars.

Side Effects of Grapefruit Seed Extract

The only known side effects of grapefruit seed extract at this time are the fact that it can increase the absorption rate of some drugs. This is because grapefruit seed extract decreases the secretion of digestive enzymes. Because of the decrease in the secretion of digestive enzymes the effect of the drug can increase.

This is particularly evident when taking drugs for hypertension and blood thinners such as Coumadin (warfarin).

It is also important to note that some commercially produced grapefruit seed extract have synthetic preparations that could possibly have side effects in some more sensitive individuals. So when first taking grapefruit seed extract you should start slow especially if you are known to be highly sensitive or allergic.

The following list will give you an idea of just how versatile grapefruit seed extract really is as a healing agent.

Here is a list of some of GSE's Internal Uses:

Acne

Allergies

Athlete's foot

Bad Breath

Benign Tumors

Bladder Infection; Interstitial

Bladder Infection; Bacterial

Blisters

Bronchitis

Candida (Fungal infection)

Candida (Vaginal Yeast)

Chronic Fatigue Syndrome

Chronic Inflammation

Colds & Flu

Corns

Coughs

Cysts

Dental Rinse

Dermatitis

Diarrhea

Dysentery

Duodenal Ulcers

Earaches

Ear Rinse

Eczema

Gas

Gastritis

Gastrointestinal Disorder

Gastrointestinal infections

Giardia lamblia -parasite

Gingivitis

Gum Disorders

Head lice

Hoarseness

Hypo-adrenal's

Hypo-tension

Insect bites & stings

Laryngitis

Lung infections

Lymph inflammation

Lymphomas

Mouthwash

Mucus Removal

Nasal Rinse

Oral Health

Parasites

Parasitic diseases

Plaque

Polyps

Psoriasis

Rashes

Respiratory infections

Runny nose

Shaving

Shingles

Sinus infections

Sore throat

Strep throat

Swollen glands

Thrush

Tonsillitis

Tooth decay

Toothaches

Tooth extraction

Toothbrush cleaner

Toxic Shock Syndrome

Ulcers

Vaginal infections

Warts

Yeast infections

GSE is a Broad Spectrum Antibiotic

Grapefruit seed extract is a wonderful broad spectrum antibiotic. It works whether you know the cause of the infection or not. Grapefruit seed extract not only kills numerous bacteria, viruses, etc. but it even boosts the function of the immune system!

So it is a wonderful resource to have on hand at any time. Imagine you are getting that blah feeling that you get when you are about to come down with the flu. Since the flu is a virus conventional antibiotics aren't an option.

What does the doctor usually tell you to do for the flu? Drink plenty of fluids and get bed rest.

Now you have another option. Taking grapefruit seed extract early enough could halt the influenza virus in its tracks. Even if you don't catch it in time grapefruit seed extract will kill the virus so it will lessen the impact of the virus while shortening its duration.

Best of all…

GSE is effective even at low concentrations.

Grapefruit seed extract is effective against over 100 types of fungi and 800 bacteria

The Journal of Alternative and Complementary Medicine 521 states that 'It was evident that grapefruit seed-extract disrupts the bacterial membrane and liberates the cytoplasmic contents within 15 minutes after contact even at more dilute concentrations '.

In 1989 researchers compared grapefruit seed extract to 30 efficient antibiotics and 18 verified fungicides. They discovered that grapefruit seed extract was found to work just as well as all of the tested agents.

Grapefruit seed extract has also been found to be nontoxic. According to a lab test "Acute Oral Toxicity" would take at least 4,000 times the normal dose to produce even a 50% chance of poisoning.

Because of how safe grapefruit seed extract is, it is becoming the natural healing choice for anyone looking for a broad spectrum agent because it doesn't have bad side effects. Besides not having bad side effects it is low cost too.

GSE is becoming a popular choice for naturopathic doctors and clinics as well as people everywhere because it doesn't have bad side effects, is low cost, easy to use and you can store a quantity that will serve you for an extended period of time in a small 4 or 8 ounce bottle.

Alkalizing For Better Health

Most degenerative diseases are connected to the pH level of their body. The pH level of your body is an important factor to look at when you are trying to conquer any serious illness or trying to maintain good health. Studies have found that most diseases cannot live in an alkaline environment. The pH level of a healthy person is usually around 7.5.

Alkalizing Vegetables

Alfalfa	Barley grass
Beet greens	Beets
Broccoli	Cabbage
Carrots	Cauliflower
Celery	Chard greens
Chlorella	Collard greens
Cucumbers	Dandelions
Dulce- a type of algae	Edible flowers
Eggplant	Fermented vegetables
Garlic	Green beans
Green peas	Kale
Kohlrabi	Lettuce
Mushrooms	Mustard greens
Nightshade vegetables	Onions
Parsnips	Peppers
Pumpkin	Radishes
Rutabaga	Sea vegetables
Spinach greens	Spirulina
Sprouts	Sweet potatoes
Tomatoes	Wheat grass
Wild Greens	

Alkalizing Fruits

Apple
Avocado
Berries
Cantaloupe
Coconut, fresh
Dates, dried
Grapes
Honeydew Melon
Lime
Nectarine
Peach
Pineapple
Raspberries
Strawberries
Tomato
Umeboshi Plums

Apricot
Banana
Blackberries
Cherries, sour
Currants
Figs, dried
Grapefruit
Lemon
Muskmelons
Orange
Pear
Raisins
Rhubarb
Tangerine
Tropical Fruits
Watermelon

Alkalizing Proteins

Almonds
Chicken Breast
Eggs (poached)
Millet
Pumpkin Seeds
Squash Seeds
Tempeh (a fermented soy)
Whey Protein Powder

Chestnuts
Cottage Cheese
Flax Seeds
Nuts
Sprouted Seeds
Sunflower Seeds
Tofu (a fermented soy)
Yogurt

Alkalizing Grains:

Amaranth	Buckwheat
Kamut	Millet
Quinoa	Spelt.

Alkalizing Spices & Seasonings

Chili Pepper	Cinnamon
Curry	Ginger
Herbs (all)	Miso
Mustard	Sea Salt
Tamari	

Alkalizing Odds & Ends

Alkaline Antioxidant Water	Apple Cider Vinegar
Bee Pollen	Fresh Fruit Juice
Green Juices	Lecithin Granules
Mineral Water	Molasses, blackstrap
Pro-biotic Cultures	Soured Dairy Products
Veggie Juices	

Some Highly Alkaline Forming Foods

Baking soda

Lemons

Lentils

Lime

Lotus root

Mineral water

Nectarine

Onion

Persimmon

Pineapple

Pumpkin seed

Raspberry

Sea salt

Sea vegetables

Seaweed

Sweet potato

Tangerine

Taro root

Watermelon

The Many Uses of Grapefruit seed extract.

Alkalizing

Grapefruit seed extract helps alkalize the body. It is considered one of the most alkaline forming foods and of all fruits it is the most alkalizing. Alkalizing the body (raising pH) is one of GSE's most important health regeneration benefits.

Matter-of-fact, lemons, limes and grapefruits are all acidic. But research has shown that when these fruits are metabolized by the body they in fact have an alkalizing effect.

There have been a growing number of people working on alkalizing their body, due in part because the typical modern diet is very acidic but also, because researchers have found that diseases are unable to live in an alkaline environment.

It has been claimed that cancer cells die in a body pH environment of 8.0. Numerous health conditions, in addition to cancer, are caused by an acidic environment. These health conditions are successfully treated by simply restoring the body to the proper pH balance.

Even though Grapefruit seed extracts' pH level is an acidic 2.0, many acidic foods actually have an alkaline effect on the body.

An acidic condition within the body is the result of eating acid forming foods such as:

Many grains

Meats

Sugars

Most degenerative diseases are thought to originate with your body's pH level. If you are trying to overcome a serious illness, or just to be able to maintain your good health, you should be looking at your PH level. Getting your body into a more alkaline state can have far reaching health benefits because the list of diseases that are caused an acidic PH level is a mile long.

It has long been believed that cancer, and most other diseases too, cannot survive an alkaline environment. The pH level of a healthy person is 7.5

Allergies

Grapefruit seed extract is an exceptional nontoxic spray for burns, cuts, insect bites, scrapes and wounds to stop infections in their tracks. GSE is tremendously beneficial in the curative process. Using grapefruit seed extract also greatly reduces any chance of re-infection.

Antibiotic

In my opinion, GSE is one of the best natural, non-toxic, antibiotics that you can have in your home.

Athlete's foot

Athlete's foot is caused by a fungus. A grapefruit seed extract solution works very well for this.

Bad Breath

Bad Breath is usually caused by bacteria running rampant inside the mouth. Tooth decay or putrefaction in the lower digestive tract can also cause bad breath otherwise known as halitosis. Grapefruit seed extract is particularly effective and a long lasting breath freshener.

Benign Tumors, Cysts, Lymphoma, Polyps, & Wens

You are supposed to be able to use grapefruit seed extract to be able to shrink Benign Tumors, Cysts, Lymphoma, Polyps, and Wens.

Mix 1-5drops of GSE in a tablespoon of carrier oil such as almond, coconut, olive or vegetable.

Rub this on 2-4 times a day.

If the growth is increasing in size then you are supposed to apply it at least 3-4 times a day.

If this concentration seems too strong and is irritating to your skin then add an extra teaspoon or two of oil if you need to.

Bladder Infection, Bacterial Cystitis and Incontinence
A frequent, urgent need to urinate and when you do it is a burning and painful urination.

Bladder Infections, Chronic Urethritis and Interstitial Cystitis

Candida infection

1st week: 1 drop taken twice a day in a cup of water
2nd week: 3 drops taken twice a day in a cup of water.
3rd week: 5-7 drops taken three times a day in a cup of water

Candida Yeast

1st week: Use 2 drops of GSE in a cup of water one time each day.

2nd week: Use 4 drops of GSE in a cup of water two times each day.

3rd week: Use 6 drops of GSE in a cup of water three times each day.

*** You can increase or decrease these doses as necessary.

Candida Yeast Infection & Vaginal Rinse

Mix 6-8 drops of GSE in a cup of warm water. Use this solution to douche one time each day for 7-10 days- or as directed by your naturopathic doctor.

Be sure that you always dilute the GSE.

For unrelenting cases it is best to douche with the solution recommended above as well as take an oral solution, of 3-7 drops in water, several times each day .

Chronic Fatigue Syndrome

Chronic fatigue syndrome is a fairly new syndrome that came about after Chernobyl.

Some people feel that it is brought about by an overload of toxins on the system.

For chronic fatigue syndrome you should take 12 drops of grapefruit seed extract in water. Drink this solution 3 times every day.

Chronic Inflammation

Chronic Inflammation is a symptom indicating that there is a weakening of the immune system which needs to be addressed.

GSE helps to boost your   immune system

Crohn's disease

There are some experts that say that many people that are diagnosed with colitis or crohn's disease are actually infected with parasites. GSE is very effective against parasites so if these experts are correct then it would be possible that grapefruit seed extract would kill said parasites and in doing so take care of the symptoms known as crohn's disease.

.Colds and Flu

Use 1-7 drops of grapefruit seed extract in a cup of water 3 times a day at the first sign of a cold or flu.

Coughs, Hoarseness and Laryngitis
Gargling with a GSE solution will help for these conditions.

Dental Caries/Tooth Decay

Dental caries is actually caused by the demineralization of the tooth enamel and the hard substance of the tooth. This is caused by the metabolic practice of plaque bacteria. Keeping teeth clean, using GSE to kill bacteria in your mouth and eating mineral rich foods can help to keep your teeth healthy and cavity-free.

Dental Rinse

Using GSE diluted in water will kill damaging oral bacteria to help to keep your mouth   healthy.

Use 1 to 5 drops grapefruit seed extract 1-2 times daily.

Diarrhea and Dysentery

Diarrhea and Dysentery are caused by bacterially contaminated food or water. Experts say that a lot of people that are diagnosed with either colitis or Crohn's disease might actually be infected with one of the following:

Amoebas

Fungi

Giardia lamblia

Parasites

Salmonella

Shigella

Grapefruit seed extract is extremely effective against these. Just be sure to start slow and to drink plenty of water because if you try to kill these off too quickly you can suffer from 'die-off' where your body has to deal with the toxins being released when these bacteria, fungus or parasites are killed.

Digestive disturbances

Many digestive issues come about due to pathogens which can be helped by the use of GSE.

Ear Infections

Take 2-7 drops diluted in water several times a day orally.

You should also mix 1 to 5 drops of GSE in 1 oz vegetable glycerin or alcohol in a dropper bottle.

When needed just put 2 to 5 drops of mixture in affected ear as often as necessary.

***Do not use full strength in ears.

Ear Rinse

A dilute solution of GSE can be used to help to keep ears clean and healthy.

Earaches

Thoroughly mix 1-5 drops GSE with 1 oz vegetable glycerin or alcohol. 1-5 drops of this mixture inserted into the affected ear several times daily should relieve most earaches.

When needed just put 2 to 5 drops of mixture in affected ear as often as necessary.

This mixture can be used as often as needed.

Do not use GSE full strength in ears.

Economical

GSE is very efficient even at low concentrations, so a little goes a long way. Most uses will only need just a few drops per dose.

A 1 oz bottle usually contains approximately 600 drops so you can see that even a one ounce bottle would last for a while.

Epstein Barr Virus

For Epstein Barr syndrome you should take 12 drops of grapefruit seed extract in water. Drink this solution 3 times every day.

External Skin Conditions

Many different types of external skin conditions, from both known and unknown causes, can be helped with grapefruit seed extract. This includes causes such as:

Bacteria

Fungal

Parasites

Viral

It is also effective to fight against fungal infections of the feet, nails and the skin.

Facial Cleanser for Oily Skin

Grapefruit seed extract is a good facial cleanser for oily skin and is quite good for fighting acne. You just need to apply 1-2 drops of GSE to your moistened fingertips and then gently massage your face in a circular motion for a minute or so. Then you rinse your face thoroughly using tepid water.

Some people have reported a tingling sensation after using the GSE treatment. This is simply a sign that the grapefruit seed extract is working.

Flatulence and Gas

Mix 1-7 drops of GSE in a cup of water. Drink this solution 3-4 times a day.

For serious gas it is recommended to take a pro-biotic each day as well as consuming a tablespoon of raw apple cider vinegar mixed in water and drink it before meals.

Instead of raw apple cider vinegar you could also use digestive enzymes.

Food sensitivities:

1 to 5 drops grapefruit seed extract 2-3 times daily.

For good health

Mix 1-7 drops of GSE in a cup of water. Drink this solution 2-4 times a day.

Fungal Infections

GSE has been found to be very effective against many types of fungal infections both internal and external.

Gastritis, Gastric and Duodenal Ulcers

Thoroughly mix 1- 5 drops of grapefruit seed extract in a cup of water. Drink 30 minutes before eating.

Do this 2 to 3 times a day until symptoms have disappeared. Then continue for an extra few days.

If your stomach is sensitive then you should start off with one drop in a cup of water. If that still bothers then you may try that strength of solution but only sip on it throughout the day so that you are getting a very dilute amount in any given time.

Then increase your dosage as needed until you get to the recommended dose.

***Note- since ulcers are very sensitive to acidic irritation care must be taken when using GSE. If the irritation persists then you should discontinue using the grapefruit seed extract as ulcers can be a very serious.

You should talk with your doctor about this issue.

Gastrointestinal Disorder

If the cause of your gastrointestinal disorder seems to be unknown then it is possible that you may be infected with:

Amoebas   Fungi

Giardia   Lamblia

Salmonella   Shigella

Or some other type of parasite that came from contaminated food, water, etc.

Mix 1-5 drops of GSE in a cup of water and drink this solution 2 times a day.

Gingivitis and Gum Disorders

Gingivitis and Gum Disorders are caused by plaque bacteria that when it is allowed to multiply can cause the gums to bleed.

 Moisten your toothbrush and apply 1 drop of GSE to it.
Brush your teeth with this solution at least twice a day. Rinse your mouth with the 'antiseptic mouthwash solution.

Hay fever

Using a preventative dose of 1-4 drops of grapefruit seed extract mixed in a cupful of water 2-3 times a day can help your body when dealing with allergies.

You may want to start this dosage ahead of known allergy seasons for you.

Use 1-4 drops in 1 cup of water 2-3 times a day

Head Lice

After using several different products for head lice some people have found relief by using grapefruit seed extract.

One person told how they used many different head lice products on their 3 year old with no results. They then tried grapefruit seed extract because they were told that it would work great for getting rid of them. After using it in their shampoo they found that the head lice were completely gone.

For anyone that works with the public, large groups of children or has kids in school you might want to consider adding some GSE to your family's shampoo as a preventative against head lice infestation.

Herpes

The Herpes virus can be stimulated by eating arginine rich foods (such as chocolate and nuts), getting too much sun as well as having too much stress.

Doctors have seen that the herpes simplex virus has become inactive, in as little as just ten minutes, after the use of grapefruit seed extract.

Thoroughly mix 2 drops of GSE with a tablespoon of olive oil and apply several times a day.

In addition it is a good idea to use GSE internally- see Antibiotic dosage in Human Uses- General Use

Hypo-adrenalism

For hypo-adrenalism you should take 12 drops of grapefruit seed extract in water. Drink this solution 3 times every day.

Hypo-tension

For hypo-tension you should take 12 drops of grapefruit seed extract in water. Drink this solution 3 times every day.

Mouthwash

Can be used as a Mouthwash for:

Fresh breath

Killing harmful bacteria and germs

Healthy gums

MRSA Infection

MRSA is a strain of the common staphylococci bacteria. It is known as Methicillin-resistant Staphylococcus aureus, or MRSA for short. MRSA is actually a much more common condition than most of us realize. It is believed that MRSA is responsible for more deaths throughout the US each year than the AIDS virus is.

It is reported that in 2005 there were 18,650 people in the US. that were killed by MRSA infections.

In the same year it is reported that AIDS killed 12,500 people.

I recently read that it is believed that around 32 out of every 100,000 US residents develop MRSA infections each year. That is 94,360 more infections than bacterial pneumonia, flesh-eating strep and meningitis combined.

These figures may be debatable but the seriousness of the MRSA infection is not. It is a very serious and dangerous infection and the MRSA bacteria are becoming resistant to our first-line of defense: antibiotic treatments.

Without effective treatment the MRSA infection can cause destruction of skin tissue which can lead to extremely painful and, very often, disfiguring abscesses. If the MRSA bacteria spread to bones, the blood stream, joints or into the vital organs then the MRSA infection can potentially cause death.

I read about a man that used GSE to cure an MSRA Infection that his mother got while she was in the hospital. His mother was dying. She had been given only a few weeks to live. This man gave his mother 5 drops of GSE twice a day. He said that in less than a week that she was getting better.

This man said that within 2 weeks his mother was cured and she was released from the hospital.

Another person told how someone he knew had a MRSA infection on his leg. MRSA is often referred to as the "flesh eating" bacteria. The person was being treated in a hospital in the Midwest. They said that the antibiotics were not doing any good. It was reported that what finally brought the MRSA infection under control was the use of Grapefruit seed extract also known as GSE.

Mucus

The production of mucous can be affected by consuming dairy products. So, if mucous is a problem it is advised that you halt consumption of all dairy products. At least until this has passed but if mucous seems to be an ongoing problem then see if avoiding dairy products for a time improves your situation.

Then slowly re-introduce dairy into your diet. In this way you can determine if dairy is an issue with you and make decisions accordingly about your diet.

Mix 1-5 drops in 1 cup water Gargle using small amounts. Repeat this several times & then drink the rest of the mixture slowly.

Parasites

Use 3-7 drops in 1 cup water taken 2-3 times a day to help to remove parasites from your system. Some parasites hide deep within your body creating health issues. For these types of parasites you will need to be vigilant and stay on this grapefruit seed extract dosage for some time.

Phlegm

Phlegm is very thick mucus. Drinking more water will help to thin it out so that it is easier to expel.

As stated previously when talking about mucous we noted that dairy could be an underlying issue.

The production of mucous can be affected by consuming dairy products. So, if mucous is a problem it is advised that you halt consumption of all dairy products. At least until this has passed but if mucous seems to be an ongoing problem then see if avoiding dairy products for a time improves your situation.

Then slowly re-introduce dairy into your diet. In this way you can determine if dairy is an issue with you and make decisions accordingly about your diet.

Mix 1-5 drops in 1 cup water Gargle using small amounts. Repeat this several times & then drink the rest of the mixture slowly.

Plaque

Plaque is a bacterial coating of the teeth that causes dental caries and periodontal gum disease. Periodontosis is a progressive gum disease.

Keeping teeth clean, using GSE to kill bacteria in your mouth and eating mineral rich foods can help to keep your teeth healthy and cavity-free

Moisten your toothbrush and apply 1 drop of GSE to it. Brush your teeth with this solution at least 3 times a day. Rinse your mouth with the 'antiseptic mouthwash' solution.

Psoriasis

Psoriasis is a skin condition that consists of dry scaly patches that itch really bad. The itching can be so intense that you itch to the point of scratching areas raw and bloody.

I know because I have been affected by this condition.

I have found that by applying a mixture of a few drops of grapefruit seed extract in some almond or olive oil and apply several times a day you can gain relief and get the patches to heal.

You could also put a few drops of GSE in a tablespoon of coconut oil and apply this to the psoriasis;

Respiratory Infections

A respiratory therapist was the first to try using grapefruit seed extract in a nebulizer. Since then, GSE has been successfully used by many people in a nebulizer to get rid of bronchial and lung infections. Most had their symptoms disappear in less than a day. Even children with chronic infections, that were unaffected by antibiotics prescribed by their doctor, were healed.

You might also be able to use the nebulizer solution in a vaporizer if you don't have a nebulizer. I don't know for sure that this would work but if you don't have a nebulizer it might be worth a try?

I have another idea for anyone who doesn't have, or can't afford, a nebulizer. You can put your nebulizer solution in a clean, empty nasile spray bottle. Then by squeezing the bottle you would inhale the mist deep into your lungs.

You would use the same solution mixture of grape fruit seed extract as you do for in a nebulizer.

Grapefruit seed extract used in a nebulizer, and the resulting vapor being inhaled, has worked for many people to get rid of bronchilal and lung infections.

For many people, using GSE in a nebulizer, their symptoms disappeared in less than 24 hours.

In one test: four of five children tested had chronic infections that had been unaffected by the antibiotics that had been prescribed by their doctor. And yet they found quick relief with nebulized grapefruit seed extract

Nebulizing grapefruit seed extract may also be effective against the sars virus, Considering the seriousness of the sars virus and how effective GSE is I would definitely try it.

This same solution may be able to be used in a vaporizer or boiling water if you don't have a nebulizer.

Skin issues: Benign Tumors, Cysts, Lymphoma, Polyps, and Wens

Mix 1 to 5 drops GSE per tablespoon of almond, avocado, olive oil, sesame or vegetable oil. Rub this medicated oil on the area 2 to 3 times daily. Three to four times a day might be necessary if the growth seems to be increasing in size.

If you find this oil is irritating to your skin then you may need to add a little more oil or reduce the amount of grapefruit seed extract. If you need to take either of these measures then you could try applying it an extra time per day.

If that extra application seems to irritate your skin then you will just have to settle for the weaker solution at the originally recommended dosage. Just so that you are aware, the treatment may take longer at the weaker dose.

Sinusitis

To use GSE as a Nasal Rinse you will need to mix 1-5 drops of GSE with 3/4 cup of tepid water.

With your head tilted back you should fill each nostril with an eyedropper full of this solution. Then, hold your breath and, quickly drop your head forward and down. Your head is now upside down which will push the solution up and into the nasal passages. Then return your head to the normal, upright position. Then just let your nasal passages drain.

IMPORTANT Do *not* inhale during this process and be sure to always dilute the GSE.

Sore Throat Gargle

Stir 1-7 drops of GSE in half a cup of water. Gargle with this solution several times a day and swallow a sip each time. You may use this solution as often as needed throughout the day but the GSE must always be diluted.

Strep Throat

Stir 1-7 drops of GSE in half a cup of water. Gargle with this solution several times a day and swallow a sip each time. You may use this solution as often as needed throughout the day but the GSE must always be diluted.

Swollen Lymph Glands (lymph Inflammation)

Lymph inflammation is an indicator that toxins are building up in that area.

Mix 1-7 drops of GSE in 4 ounces of water. Use this solution to gargle with several times a day.

It would also be a good idea to take either the maintenance dose or antibiotic dose internally depending on how you feel

Tonsillitis

Stir 1-7 drops of GSE in half a cup of water. Gargle with this solution several times a day and swallow a sip each time. You may use this solution as often as needed throughout the day but the GSE must always be diluted.

Thrush

Thrush is actually a fungal infection of the mouth. It is recognized by the white coating found in the mouth. Thrush is caused by a yeast fungus known as Candida Albicans or Candida for short.

Rinse the mouth well 3-4 times a day with 4-6 drops of GSE in 8 ounces of water.

Toothaches

Mix 1 to 5 drops grapefruit seed extract in 1cup of water and gargle with this several times each day. You can also soak a cotton pad in a solution of 1 to 5 drops grapefruit seed extract mixed into 2-4 ounces of water. Place the soaked cotton pad directly on the aching tooth. This will help for pain while killing germs to enhance healing of any infection that is present and is causing the pain.

Toothache oil

Another option is to get your self a clean bottle, either with a squeeze top or a dropper, to mix up a toothache relieving/infection fighting oil.

Fill your bottle with pure virgin olive oil. Organic is best. If your bottle is 1 ounce then you can add 5-15 drops of grapefruit seed extract. Mix well. You can apply a drop or two of this mixture to your finger and rub it on the affected gum area or drip a drop or two directly onto the tooth.

Use this in addition to the GSE that you ingest for infection.

Tooth Extraction

In order to relieve pain you should use 1 to 5 drops grapefruit seed extract in 1 cup of water and use this to gargle with and you can take 5-10 drops of grapefruit seed extract in 20 ounces of juice, pop, tea, water, etc. Take this several times a day. Drinking fluids with grapefruit seed extract in them will work to prevent and heal infection.

Toothbrush Cleaner

WOW! Did you know that it has been reported that up to 1 million bacteria can live on your toothbrush.

When you have a cold or flu do you thoroughly clean your toothbrush or replace it?

Well now you know that you can use grapefruit seed extract to clean your toothbrush as it kills bacteria, viruses and pretty much anything that could be found on your toothbrush that could possibly make you sick.

Check out the upcoming section that tells the doses for different uses and you will find out how you can safely disinfect your family's toothbrushes.

Toxic Shock Syndrome

As a preventive measure, when you use tampons, it is a good idea to douche using a solution of 1-7 drops of GSE diluted in a quart of warm water.

Ulcers

Ulcerative Stomatitis is a contagious disease. It causes the throat and tongue to become red, swollen and extremely sore. Ulcerative Stomatitis may affect the inside area of the cheeks, as well as the lips and palate. It can also create inflamed gums that will bleed easily.

Urinary issues

Bladder infection

Chronic urethritis

Interstitial cystitis

Virulent Staphylococci Infection

GSE works well against staphylococci infection. If it is a virulent staphylococci infection you would probably want to increase your dosage strength as well as frequency.

It may take a while if the infection is very bad then it may take a while but keep at it. The great thing with GSE is the fact that you can safely take it at fairly high doses and for long periods of time.

I have and I have only positive things to say about GSE. I have never had a bad reaction.

The worst thing that happened to me was at the high doses I started to have a loose stool and so I cut back on my dose.

Weight loss

GSE is a very powerful antioxidant. It helps people to lose weight because it stimulates your metabolism. It also helps the body to operate more efficiently because it decreases the toxins in your body.

These toxins are created from stress, environmental aspects and from your dietary habits.

Because it destroys these toxins it decreases cortisol production. Cortisol is a strong inhibitor of the hormones T3 and T4. These hormones control a large portion pf your metabolism. GSE also increases your digestion, reduces cholesterol, helps your body to use nutrients better and it helps to promote better health.

These all help to maintain your proper body weight.

Personally, I have found that since I have been using GSE on a regular basis that I don't gain weight so easily and I have slowly went down a couple of sizes without being on a diet or cutting out treats.

Wounds

Grapefruit seed extract is an exceptional nontoxic spray for burns, cuts, insect bites, scrapes and wounds to stop infections in their tracks. GSE is tremendously beneficial in the curative process. Using grapefruit seed extract also greatly reduces any chance of re-infection.

Doses for Numerous Health Conditions

All doses can be taken with or without food and can be mixed in:

Juice   Pop

Tea   Water

So, for reference, whenever I mention to mix the GSE in water it can be mixed in any of these fluids EXCEPT when it is to be used to gargle or apply to a wound. In those cases it should only be mixed with water.

Basic dose is usually as follows:

Adults- 5-15 drops of GSE in a glass of water 1-3 times a day.

Children (5 years and older)- 1-3 drops in a glass of water 1-2 times a day..

For internal use a good rule of thumb is to use one drop of liquid concentrate for every 10 pounds of body weight.

Alkalizing

Simply using a few drops of grapefruit seed extract a day will help to counteract the acidity in your body.

Of course the more acidic your body is the more alkalinity you need to offset the acidity. In other words the more acidic your body PH level the more you need to alkalize. Not only is using a maintenance dose of GSE great for alkalizing but you should also be getting alkalizing foods into your diet:.

See Alkalizing Foods section for more information on alkalizing your system for better health.

Allergies

Using a preventative dose of 1-4 drops of grapefruit seed extract mixed in a cupful of water 2-3 times a day can help your body when dealing with allergies.

You may want to start this dosage ahead of known allergy seasons for you.

Antibiotic

Mix 5-10 drops of grapefruit seed extract in 1 cup of water 3-5 times a day. This dose can be increased or decreased when necessary.

Bad Breath

Rinse your mouth, and also gargle with, a solution using 1 to 5 drops grapefruit seed extract in 1 cup water at least 3 times a day. You can do this as often as you feel necessary.

If you believe that the bad breath begins in the digestive tract, rather than it being caused by a dental issue, then you should drink 1 to 5 drops of grapefruit seed extract mixed in 1/2 cup of fluid 2-3 times a day.

If you are unsure of the underlying cause of the bad breath then it would be a good idea to rinse *and* use the dose for digestive issues.

Bladder Infection, Bacterial Cystitis and Incontinence

These types of infections are known to have the following symptoms:

Burning urination

Frequent urination

Painful urination

Urgent urination

It is important that as soon as you feel any of these symptoms that you should start to take a few drops of grapefruit seed extract and 1 teaspoon of baking soda in 1 cup of water. You should drink this solution three times each day and continue taking this for 7-10 days.

Candida Fungal Infections

1st week:

Use 2 drops of GSE in a cup of water one time each day.

2nd week:

Use 4 drops of GSE in a cup of water two times each day.

3rd week:

Use 6 drops of GSE in a cup of water three times each day.

*** You can increase or decrease these doses as necessary.

Candida Yeast Infections Vaginal Rinse

Use 8 drops of GSE in a of cup water, mix well and use this to douche one time each day for a week (or as directed by your doctor).

You must always be sure to dilute the grapefruit seed extract before using.

If your candida yeast infection is relentless then you should take the internal dose recommended above at the same time as using the douche remedy.

Chronic Fatigue Syndrome

12 drops grapefruit seed extract. Drink this solution 3 times daily.

Chronic Inflammation

Use 12 drops of GSE in a cup of water 2-3 times each day. You can increase this dose if necessary.

Colds and Flu

Use 1-7 drops of grapefruit seed extract. Drink this solution 3 times each day at the first sign of a cold or flu. The sooner you start this the better the results for stopping the cold or flu in its tracks. At the very least it should reduce the length and the severity of your illness.

Coughs, Hoarseness and Laryngitis

Use 1-6 drops of GSE in a cup of water. Gargle with this solution 3-5 times each day.

It is recommended that you either:

Swallow a mouthful or two of this solution every time that you gargle. This will help you to heal faster.

OR

Use 2-7 drops of GSE in a cup of water and drink a cup of this 2-3 times a day.

Dental Caries & Tooth Decay

Use a drop of GSE on a moist toothbrush to brush your teeth 3 times a day. After you brush your teeth it is a good idea to rinse your mouth with a solution of 4 drops of GSE in a cup of water.

For more rigorous cases you can put 4-6 drops of GSE in 1/4 cup of water. Moisten a bit of cotton or gauze and place it on your gums for several minutes a day.

Dental Rinse

1 to 5 drops grapefruit seed extract mixed in a half of a cup of water. Rinse with this solution 1-2 times daily.

Diarrhea and Dysentery

1 to 5 drops grapefruit seed extract in a cup of water. Drink this solution 1-2 times a day. This solution can also be used as a preventative measure if you drink it each day.

Ear Rinse and Earaches

Be sure to thoroughly mix 2-5 drops of GSE in 1 oz of vegetable glycerin or alcohol in a dropper bottle.

Squeeze 2-5 drops of this mixture in affected ear several times a day or as often as needed. *Never* use GSE full strength in your ears.

Epstein Barr Virus

Mix 10-12 drops of grapefruit seed extract in a cup of water. Drink this solution 3 times daily.

Flatulence and Gas

Use 1-5 drops of GSE in a cup of water. Drink this 3 times a day. A pro-biotic can help to replenish your beneficial bacteria to help to minimize this problem.

Food sensitivities:

1 to 5 drops grapefruit seed extract 2-3 times daily.

Gastritis, Gastric and Duodenal Ulcers

1-5 drops GSE in a cup of water

Drink this solution 30 minutes before your meal. Do this 2-3 times a day. Continue this dosage until your symptoms are gone.

If you have a sensitive stomach then you should start off with just 1-5 drops of GSE and then increase the dosage as necessary. The more sensitive your stomach the smaller the initial dosage should be.

WARNING

Ulcers can be very sensitive to acidity. So care should be taken when you use GSE. If irritation continues then you should stop using the grapefruit seed extract since having ulcers can be a serious condition. It is recommended that you talk with your doctor.

Gastrointestinal Disorder

1-6 drops of GSE in a cup of water and drink this solution 2 times a day.

Gingivitis and Gum Disorders

Mix 1-7 drops of GSE in a half of a cup of water. Use this solution to moisten your toothbrush and then brush your teeth thoroughly 3 times a day.

Then, rinse your mouth with the remaining solution. For more severe cases you can use 2-7 drops of GSE in 2 ounces of warm water. Use this to moisten a piece of cotton, or gauze, and then leave it on your gums for 5-10 minutes each day.

Lungs

GSE Cough Medicine

1 ½ oz raw honey

1 ½ oz raw apple cider vinegar

50 drops GSE

½ oz vegetable glycerine

Mix ingredients until they are all incorporated. Shake well before each use. Take a Tablespoon 3-5 times daily at the beginning of chronic bronchitis, colds, sore throat, etc.

Your cough should clear up in a matter of just a few days but you should continue to take the GSE for at least a week to 10 days. If you stop taking the SE too soon then remaining bacteria would have an opportunity to multiply

You can also use GSE effectively in a nebulizer in order to create a healing mist that will coat the inside of your lungs and will then heal your bronchial and lung infections. We have even had our lungs heal after taking antibiotics without much success. Our lungs improved in just a day or two with the GSE mist.

Orally

Thoroughly mix 2-5 drops of GSE in a cup of water. Drink this solution 2-3 times a day.

For over all good health

Mix 1-7 drops of GSE in a cup of water and drink this solution 3-4 times a day.

Hay fever

1 to 5 drops grapefruit seed extract 2-3 times daily.

Head Lice

After using several different products for head lice some people have found relief by using grapefruit seed extract.

One person told how they used many different head lice products on their 3 year old with no results. They then tried grapefruit seed extract because they were told that it would work great for getting rid of them. After using it in their shampoo they found that the head lice were completely gone.

For anyone that works with the public, large groups of children or has kids in school you might want to consider adding some GSE to your family's shampoo as a preventative against head lice infestation.

Add 7-10 drops of GSE to your family's bottle of shampoo. This can be used as a preventative or to fight against head lice infestation.

Hypo-adrenalism

12 drops grapefruit seed extract. Drink this solution 3 times daily.

Hypo-tension

12 drops grapefruit seed extract. Drink this solution 3 times daily.

MRSA Infection

Take 5 drops of GSE 2-3 times a day internally.

You should also mix 5-10 drops of grapefruit seed extract in 1 cup of distilled water in a new, clean spray bottle and use this to spray the infected area several times each day.

Mouthwash:

1 to 5 drops grapefruit seed extract in 1 cup water and then vigorously swish a mouthful for about 10 seconds. Do this 1-2 times daily.

Alternatively you can add 1-5 drops of GSE to the reserve of your mouth cleansing device.

***This should be used only for adults and children over 7 years old.

Mucus Removal

1 to 7 drops grapefruit seed extract in 1-cup water and gargle deep in the throat. Repeat this several times and then slowly drink what is left in the cup.

Parasites

1 to 5 drops grapefruit seed extract 2-3 times daily

For internal use. Mix (?) drops grapefruit seed extract in 1 cup water or juice. 2-3 times daily. If you have a sensitive stomach take after meals until stomach adjusts to the extract and then you can take it independent of meals. Doses can be increased or decreased as necessary.

Phlegm Removal

1 to 7 drops grapefruit seed extract in 1-cup water and gargle deep in the throat. Repeat this several times and then slowly drink what is left in the cup.

Plaque:

1 to 7 drops grapefruit seed extract in 1-cup water and gargle deep in the throat. Repeat this several times and then slowly drink what is left in the cup.

It would also be a good idea to put 1-4 drops of grapefruit seed extract in 4 ounces of water, mix well, and then rinse your mouth thoroughly.

Respiratory Infection

1 drop in 1 ounce saline solution in nebulizer for lung infections

Sinusitis and Nasal Rinse

To use GSE as a Nasal Rinse you will need to mix 1-6 drops of GSE with 3/4 cup of tepid water.

With your head tilted back you should fill each nostril with an eyedropper full of this solution. Then, hold your breath and, quickly drop your head forward and down. Your head is now upside down which will push the solution up and into the nasal passages. Then return your head to the normal, upright position. Then just let your nasal passages drain.

IMPORTANT Do *not* inhale during this process and be sure to always dilute the GSE.

Skin issues: Benign Tumors, Cysts, Lymphoma, Polyps, Skin tags and sebaceous cysts

Mix 1 to 5 drops GSE per tablespoon of almond, avocado, olive oil, sesame or vegetable oil. Rub this medicated oil on the area 2 to 3 times daily. Three to four times a day might be necessary if the growth seems to be increasing in size.

If you find this oil is irritating to your skin then you may need to add a little more oil or reduce the amount of grapefruit seed extract. If you need to take either of these measures then you could try applying it an extra time per day.

If that extra application seems to irritate your skin then you will just have to settle for the weaker solution at the originally recommended dosage. Just so that you are aware, the treatment may take longer at the weaker dose.

Types of sore throat:

Sore Throat

Strep Throat,

Swollen Glands (lymph Inflammation)

Tonsillitis

Mix 1-7 drops of GSE in 4 ounces of water. Use this solution to gargle with several times a day. This can be used as often as needed of your throat is extremely sore. Just be sure to always dilute the GSE before use.

If you don't start feeling better within 24-48 hours then you can increase the dosage if you feel it is necessary for improvement.

Thrush

Rinse the mouth about 3 times daily with 1 to 5 drops grapefruit seed extract in 1 cup of water.

Toothaches

Mix 1 to 5 drops grapefruit seed extract in 1cup of water and gargle with this several times each day. You can also soak a cotton pad in a solution of 1 to 5 drops grapefruit seed extract mixed into

2-4 ounces of water. Place the soaked cotton pad directly on the aching tooth. This will help for pain while killing germs to enhance healing of any infection present that is causing the pain.

Tooth Extraction

In order to relieve pain you should use 1 to 5 drops grapefruit seed extract in 1cup of water and use this to gargle with and you can take 5-10 drops of grapefruit seed extract in 20 ounces of juice, pop, tea, water, etc. Drinking fluids with grapefruit seed extract in them will work to prevent and heal infection.

Toothbrush Cleaner

Mix 1-5 drops of GSE in a cup of water and let your toothbrush sit in this solution for 15-20 minutes.

You can mix this solution fresh every few days and just leave your toothbrush in it between brushings. Just be sure to rinse your toothbrush before each use.

Researchers have discovered that up to 1 million bacteria can live on your toothbrush. So, it is important to keep your toothbrush clean. This is especially important whenever you are sick with a cold, flu or anything else where the bacteria could stay alive on your toothbrush and keep re-infecting you.

Toxic Shock Syndrome

If you regularly use tampons then you may be concerned about Toxic Shock Syndrome which is a rare but hazardous disease.

As a preventive measure, when you use tampons, it is a good idea to douche using a solution of 1-7 drops of GSE diluted in a quart of warm water.

Ulcers

Mix 1-9 drops of GSE in a cup of lukewarm water. Use this solution to rinse your mouth by gargling with it several times each day and swallow a small amount each time.

Safety measure

You should make sure to sterilize your toothbrush after each use in order to keep from spreading bacteria from one use to the next.

Urinary issues

Mix 3-5 drops of GSE in a cup of water and drink this solution 3 times a day for 30 days.

Virulent Staphylococci Infection

Mix 10-12 drops of grapefruit seed extract in a cup of water. Drink this solution 3-5 times a day.

Continue this dosage for at least 7-10 days or longer if necessary.

Wounds

Grapefruit seed extract is an extraordinary non-toxic spray that can be used for:

Burns	Cuts
Insect bites	Scrapes
Wounds	

Use a mixture of 10 drops of GSE in 4 ounces of water, mix well and keep in a spray bottle. Spray this solution on wounds in order to stop infections in their tracks.

GSE is extremely helpful in the healing process. Using GSE also significantly reduces the chance of re-infection.

Some Other GSE Benefits

Alkalizes blood
Biodegradable
Broad Spectrum germ killer
Derived from natural sources
Long-term use has no negative side effects
Minimal short-term impact on beneficial bacteria
Non toxic
Powerful and effective
Supplies vitamins and minerals

Well researched

Herxheimer Reaction – Detox Response

You may wonder what the Herxheimer Reaction is?

A 'Herxheimer reaction' is basically a detoxification response. The 'Herxheimer reaction' is named after the Austrian dermatologist brothers Jarisch Adolf Herxheimer and Karl Herxheimer.

In the late 1800's the Herxheimer brothers discovered this reaction was the result of toxins that were being released as microbes died off. This created an influx of immense quantities of microbial waste.

This toxic waste created from the microbial die off interferes with the body's ability to efficiently eliminate these toxins through the usual means. Since the liver, kidney's and colon are overwhelmed the burden of all of these toxins the body is forced to eliminate them by other means.

When this happens these wastes are then released through the lungs, sinuses and even the skin.

When the Herxheimer Reaction occurs there is a 'flu-like condition' with the following symptoms:

Diarrhea

Fever (with or without chills)

Flushing

Headaches

Heavy perspiration and night sweats

Itching

Malaise

Nausea and vomiting

Pain in joints and bones

Rashes or skin lesions

Sore muscles

Usually, the Herxheimer reaction starts to manifest within 24 hours or even days or weeks after you start using GSE. The intensity of the healing crisis is relative to the body's toxicity level.

These symptoms are only temporary and show you that there was infection there. It also shows you that the treatment is working.

Alkalizing the Blood

Researchers have found that there is another important benefit of using GSE. That is the fact that it is helpful in alkalizing the blood. By raising the PH of the body you can reap numerous important health restoration benefits. Since disease causing bacteria, fungi, viruses, etcetera cannot survive in an alkaline oxygenated environment it is a good idea to try to keep your body in a more alkaline state.

Besides using GSE you can incorporate lemons, limes and grapefruit into your diet since, even though they are an acidic fruit, they have an alkalizing effect on the body.

But achieving alkalinity is not just about eating lemons and limes. It is important that you get more fresh fruits and vegetables into your diet on a daily basis. Most fruits and vegetables are alkaline forming.

Candida Yeast & Parasitic Infections

GSE works great, as well as being very safe and works without devastating side effects.

In regards to treatment GSE seems to be as effective as caprylic acid, nystatin and other common anti-fungal medications. Some doctors even believe that GSE is a 'major therapeutic breakthrough for patients with chronic parasitic and yeast infections'. And GSE seems to be much better tolerated by sensitive individuals than other antifungal treatments. GSE has been tolerated by some people when no other medication was tolerated or even worked for them.

In test results regarding 20 women with vaginal yeast infections it was found that by simply douching with a GSE solution every 12 hours that 15 of the women found relief after just 3 days.

Natural Methods to Release Toxins

Make sure to drink at least 6-8 glasses of clean, chlorine-free, water every day. This will help assist in detoxification by flushing out toxins.

Fasting

Fasting is a good way to release toxins. Keep your diet light to avoid constipation.
Consume 1-2 Tablespoons of ground flax each day in a cup of milk or diluted juice.

You should start slow, with just a teaspoon of ground flax daily and increase this until you are taking 1-2 tablespoons a day.

Hydrogen Peroxide Therapy – Soak your feet each day in

warm water with 1 cup of Hydrogen Peroxide for 30 minutes to help to draw out toxins.

Moderate exercise such as going for a walk for 30 minutes or spend 15-30 minutes on a mini-trampoline.

Rebounding not only helps to release toxins but will actually help to
Cleanse your lymph glands.

Sauna

Making use of a sauna, or hot baths, cam help your body to excrete toxins through your largest eliminatory organ- your skin.

Make sure not to overdo it or you can get light headed and could pass out. Taking short saunas more often is a much better idea rather than taking long saunas. This will also release toxins on a regular basis which will help to clear your body of toxins without the shock of a sudden large cleanse.

Charts for the uses of GSE

Human Uses- General Use	
Maintenance dose- to stay healthy	3-5 drops mixed in 1 cup water 2-3 times a day
Allergies	1-4 drops in 1 cup water 2-3 times a day
Antibiotic	4-10 drops in 1 cup water 3 times a day. This dose can be increased or decreased as necessary.
Candida infection	1st week: 1 drop taken twice a day in a cup of water 2nd week: 3 drops taken twice a day in a cup of water. 3rd week: 5-7 drops taken three times a day in a cup of water
Chronic inflammation	2-7 drops in 1 cup water 2-3 times a day
Colds & flu (influenza)	3-5 drops in 1 cup water taken 2-3 times a day

Chronic fatigue or epstein barr virus'	3-7 drops in 1 cup water taken 3 times a day
Benign tumors, cysts, etc.	20- 30 drops GSE in 1 Tablespoon of olive oil. Rub this medicated oil the affected area on 2 or 3 times a day

Bronchitis, lung & respiratory infections	1 drop GSE in 1-2 ounces of distilled water in a nebulizer and use natural cough medicine recipe listed in this book
Parasites	3-7 drops in 1 cup water taken 2-3 times a day
Mucous & phlegm removal	1-5 drops in 1 cup water Gargle using small amounts. Repeat this several times & then drink the rest of the solution slowly.
Surgery	Take the maintenance dosage

	for at least 3-7 days before your surgery and then continue it for another week or so after
Diarrhea or Dysentery	2 -7 drops in 1 cup water taken 2-3 times a day

Human Gastric & Intestinal Disorders	
Flatulence (gas)	3-7 drops in 1 cup water taken 3 times a day
Gastrointestinal disorders	2-5 drops in 1 cup water taken 2 times daily
Gastritis & ulcers	1-5 drops to 1-cup water taken 30 minutes before eating. Do this 2 to 3 times a day until your symptoms are gone

***Those with a sensitive stomach must start, and gradually increase, much more slowly.

If the irritation persists discontinue use and consult a Dr. as ulcers can cause serious bleeding. |

Human Ears, Nose & Throat	
Coughs	3-5 drops in 1 cup lukewarm water, use to gargle 3-5 times a day.
Ear rinse	1-3 drops with 1 oz. vegetable glycerin or alcohol. Use 1-2 drops of this mixture in affected ears several times a day. **NEVER** use full strength GSE in your ears.
Earache	1-3 drops with 1 oz. vegetable glycerin or alcohol. Use 1-2 drops of this mixture in affected ears several times a day. **NEVER** use full strength GSE in your ears
Hoarseness	3-5 drops in 1 cup lukewarm water, use to gargle 3-5 times a day.

Laryngitis	3-5 drops in 1 cup lukewarm water, use to gargle 3-5 times a day.
Nasal rinse	Mix 1-6 drops of GSE with 3/4 cup of tepid water. See dosage section for further instructions
Sinusitis	Mix 1-6 drops of GSE with 3/4 cup of tepid water. See dosage section for further instructions
Sore throat	Mix 1-7 drops of GSE in 4 ounces of water. Use this solution to gargle with several times a day.
Strep throat	Mix 1-7 drops of GSE in 4 ounces of water. Use this solution to gargle with several times a day.
Swollen glands (lymph inflammation)	Mix 1-7 drops of GSE in 4 ounces of water. Use this solution to gargle

	with several times a day. It would also be a good idea to take either the maintenance dose or antibiotic dose internally depending on how you feel
Human Bladder / Yeast Infections	
Bacterial cystitis	Mix 3-7 drops of GSE and 1 teaspoon of baking soda in a cup of water and drink this solution 3 times a day.
Candida	Mix 1-3 drops in a cup of water. Douche one time each day for 7-9 days. Be sure to always dilute the GSE.
Chronic Urethritis	Mix 3-7 drops of GSE in a cup of water and drink this solution 3 times a day for 30 days

Incontinence	Mix 3-7 drops of GSE and 1 teaspoon of baking soda in a cup of water and drink this solution 3 times a day.
Interstial cystitis	Mix 3-7 drops of GSE in a cup of water and drink this solution 3 times a day for 30 days
Toxic shock syndrome	Tampon use can trigger a staph or strep infection you should douche with 3-4 drops of GSE in a quart of warm water.
Vaginal douche	Mix 1-3 drops in a cup of water. Douche one time each day for 7-9 days. Be sure to always dilute the GSE.

Yeast infection	Mix 1-3 drops in a cup of water. Douche one time each day for 7-9 days. Be sure to always dilute the GSE.

Human Uses- Internal	
Antiseptic mouthwash	Mix 2-4 drops of GSE into 8 ounces of water. Briskly swish a small amount of this solution around in your mouth for 20-30 seconds. Then spit it out. Do this a couple of times a day You can add a drop of GSE to your "Waterpik" Reservoirs Only for people over six years old.
Bad breath	Gargle with a solution of 4-6 drops of GSE in

	8 ounces of water 2-3 times daily. If the underlying issue is the digestive track then you should ingest 3-5 drops of GSE mixed in 8 ounces of water several times a day.
Bleeding gums	Moisten your toothbrush and apply 1 drop of GSE to it. Brush your teeth with this solution at least twice a day. Rinse your mouth with the 'antiseptic mouthwash' solution.
Gingivitis	Moisten your toothbrush and apply 1 drop of GSE to it. Brush your teeth with this solution at least twice a day. Rinse your mouth with the 'antiseptic mouthwash' solution.
Gum disorders	Moisten your toothbrush and apply 1 drop of GSE to it. Brush your teeth with this solution at least twice a day. Rinse your mouth with the 'antiseptic mouthwash' solution. For severe cases, mix 3-5 drops of GSE into 2-4 oz water, soak a cotton (or gauze) pad with this

	solution and place it on the gums, for several minutes each day.
Plaque	Moisten your toothbrush and apply 1 drop of GSE to it. Brush your teeth with this solution at least 3 times a day. Rinse your mouth with the 'antiseptic mouthwash' solution.
Thrush- yeast fungus	Rinse the mouth well 3-4 times a day with 4-6 drops of GSE in 8 ounces of water.
Tooth aches	Gargle with mix of **3-4** drops in **1 cup** water several times daily. In addition, place cotton pad soaked in a mix of **1** drop in **2-4oz** water directly on the aching tooth.
Tooth decay	Moisten your toothbrush and apply 1 drop of GSE to it. Brush your teeth with this solution at least twice a day. Rinse your mouth with the 'antiseptic mouthwash' solution. For severe cases, mix 3-5 drops of GSE into 2-4 oz

	water, soak a cotton (or gauze) pad with this solution and place it on the gums, for several minutes each day.
Tooth extraction	Gargle with a solution of 3-5 drops of GSE in 8 ounces of lukewarm water.
Ulcers	Thoroughly mix 3-4 drops of GSE in 8 ounces of lukewarm water. Gargle and vigorously rinse your mouth several times each day. To arrest the development of this condition you should sanitize your toothbrush often.

Human Uses-		
External		
Acne	Use the facial cleaner listed below. Chronic acne-Dilute 2-3 drops of GSE in 8 ounces of water. Drink this solution 3-4 times a day.	
Athlete's foot	In a spray bottle mix 20-25 drops of GSE into 16 ounces of water. Be sure to generously spray this solution twice daily for at least 3 weeks- doing so on *clean* feet.	

		Use 20 drops of GSE to each small (or 40 drops of GSE for a large) load, last rinse cycle, of socks. Be sure to allow socks to soak for 10-15 minutes in order to avoid re-infecting your feet Spray inside of your shoes thoroughly. For serious cases: moisten feet with water, then rub in 3-5 drops of GSE and work into a lather. Let sit 2-3 minutes and rinse thoroughly.
s	Blister	Apply **1** drop on the blisters to disinfect.
	Body wash	To keep your skin clean without toxins you simply squeeze a few drops of GSE to a sponge and wash your body. Be careful that you **do not get in your eyes**.
es	Callus	Soak your feet for 10 minutes in 20-22 drops of GSE for every gallon of warm water. This removes this hard skin.
n	Chicke pox	Thoroughly mix 3 drops of GSE with a tablespoon of olive oil. Apply this to the affected areas of the skin. Alternatively you can mix 3-6 drops of GSE into 8 ounces of water and spray this solution onto the affected area when needed. In addition it is a good idea to

	use GSE internally- see Antibiotic dosage in Human Uses- General Use
Cold sores- Herpes Simplex Virus	Thoroughly mix 2 drops of GSE with a tablespoon of olive oil. In addition it is a good idea to use GSE internally- see Antibiotic dosage in Human Uses- General Use The Herpes virus can be stimulated by eating arginine rich foods (such as chocolate and nuts), getting too much sun and having too much stress.
Corns	Apply a drop of GSE full strength onto the corn a couple of times a day.
Cracked or sunburned lips	Mix a couple of drops of GSE into a tablespoon of coconut oil in shortening for a solid version you can keep in a tin or an old lip balm container/ Or you can mix a couple of drops in a tablespoon of olive (or vegetable) oil. Apply several times a day.
Dandruff	Add 3-4 drops of GSE to a handful of your favorite shampoo and mix it together while lathering up your wet hair. Massage it into your

	scalp and leave on for 3-5 minutes and then rinse it out. For in between shampooings you can mix 3-4 drops of GSE in 8 ounces of water in a spray bottle. Spray your scalp well and then rub this solution into your scalp and let it dry. **Do not get it in your eyes.**
Deodorant- Non-toxic	Mix 15-20 drops of GSE in 16 ounces of water in a spray bottle. Shake well before each use. Spray under arms.
Eczema	Mix 6-8 drops of GSE with 4 ounces of coconut or olive oil. Apply this and gently rub it into the affected area 2-3 times a day. Try to ascertain & eliminate the offending chemicals or chemicals. Use natural soaps.
Facial cleanser	Dampen your face and hands with warm water. Apply a couple of drops of GSE to your fingertips and gently massage your entire face being careful not to get it in your eyes. Then rinse your face well and pat it dry. You may feel a slight tingling sensation which indicates that

		it is deep cleaning your skin.
Head lice		Mix a tablespoon of GSE into a couple of tablespoons of shampoo. Spread this over every bit of your hair & scalp. Cover the entire head of hair with a plastic bag. Leave this on for 30-45 minutes and then rinse well. Repeat this procedure again in 3 days. **Do not get it in your eyes.**
	Hives	Thoroughly mix 3-4 drops of GSE with a tablespoon of either coconut or olive oil (depending on if you prefer a more solid, or liquid, version). Apply to affected area of your skin several times daily. Or you can mix 4-5 drops of GSE in a spray bottle filled with 8 ounces of water and mist the affected area often.
Impeti go		Mix a teaspoon of GSE to 3-4 ounces of water in a clean spray bottle and spray this solution on the affected area several times a day. Benefit has been found by adding a teaspoon of Marigold (Calendula Officianlis) to this solution.

		To decontaminate clothing, towels, etc, you can add 20 drops of GSE to the rinse cycle for a small load (and 40 drops for a large load). Allow the load to soak for a while. Before finishing rinse cycle
Insect bites		Apply a drop of undiluted GSE. If this irritates the skin then mix a drop of GSE in a spoonful of coconut oil and apply as needed to insect bites.
Leeches		Put a drop or two of GSE directly on the leech. Wait a minute or two and then remove the leech. Apply another drop of GSE directly on the bite in order to disinfect it to avoid infection.
Nail treatment		Mix 2-3 drops of GSE into a tablespoon of water or grain alcohol such as vodka. Rub into your nails and cuticles a generous amount of this solution. Do this a couple of times a day. Nail fungus is quite resistant so you will have to be persistent as it could take a few months of regular use. For particularly stubborn cases you can add more drops of GSE. You can use the GSE full strength if it is necessary to eradicate the fungus. It might also be a good idea to ingest the antibiotic dose.
Poison ivy		In a spray bottle mix 2 teaspoons of GSE in 10 tablespoons of water. Apply to a small test area on affected area of the skin.

		If it burns, or seems irritated, then add a little water and shake well. Spray the affected area generously with this solution and repeat every couple of hours or as needed. Shake well before each use.
	Poison oak	In a spray bottle mix 2 teaspoons of GSE in 10 tablespoons of water. Apply to a small test area on affected area of the skin. If it burns, or seems irritated, then add a little water and shake well. Spray the affected area generously with this solution and repeat every couple of hours or as needed. Shake well before each use..
Psorias is		Twice a day rub the affected areas with a mixture of 4 drops of GSE in 2 ounces of coconut or olive oil.
	Rashes	Thoroughly mix 3-4 drops of GSE with a tablespoon of either coconut or olive oil (depending on if you prefer a more solid, or liquid, version). Apply to affected area of your skin several times daily. Or you can mix 4-5 drops of GSE in a spray bottle

		filled with 8 ounces of water and mist the affected area often.
Ringw orm		In a spray bottle, mix a teaspoon of GSE to 2-3 ounces of water. Generously spray the affected area. If it burns, or seems irritated, then add a little water and shake well. Spray the affected area generously with this solution and repeat every couple of hours or as needed. Shake well before each use. You can use olive or coconut oil instead of water. Apply to the affected area twice a day. Continue using for 7-10 days after the symptoms are gone in order to be sure that the skin fungus has died. Treat all the affected areas at the same time and let the area get fresh air and sunshine. **Do not get in your eyes**.
	Shavin g rash	Add 2-3 drops of GSE to your shaving cream; You can use the GSE facial cleanser listed above as an aftershave. Be sure to sterilize your razor and the blades before and after each use
Shingl es		Mix a few drops of GSE in a tablespoon of coconut or olive

	oil. You should apply this to the skin several times a day. Another method is to mix 4-5 drops of GSE in 8 ounces of water. Mix well and generously spray the affected area as often as needed.
Skin fungi	In a spray bottle, mix a teaspoon of GSE to 2-3 ounces of water. Generously spray the affected area. If it burns, or seems irritated, then add a little water and shake well. Spray the affected area generously with this solution and repeat every couple of hours or as needed. Shake well before each use. You can use olive or coconut oil instead of water. Apply to the affected area twice a day. Continue using for 7-10 days after the symptoms are gone in order to be sure that the skin fungus has died. Treat all the affected areas at the same time and let the area get fresh air and sunshine. **Do not get in your eyes**.
Stinging nettle rash	.Thoroughly mix 3-4 drops of GSE with a tablespoon of either coconut or olive oil (depending on if you prefer a more solid, or liquid, version). Apply to affected area

	of your skin several times daily. Or you can mix 4-5 drops of GSE in a spray bottle filled with 8 ounces of water and mist the affected area often.
Stings	Apply GSE in an undiluted form. If the skin is sensitive, mix with a little bit of water or olive oil.
Ticks	Put a drop or two of GSE directly on the tick. Wait a minute or two and then remove the tick. Apply another drop of GSE directly on the bite in order to disinfect it to avoid infection. If you live in an infested area be sure to thoroughly check for deer ticks, Deer ticks can transmit Ehrlichia, which is a serious pathogen that causes HGE (human granulocytic ehrlichiosis) a sometimes fatal disease As a preventative measure you can drink 8-10 drops of GSE mixed in a cup of water 3-4 times a day for a couple of weeks.

Varicose veins	Mix 8-10 drops of GSE in 4 ounces of cooled, boiled water. Dampen a clean cotton, or gauze, pad. Place on the effected area. Keep the pad moist and renew it often.
Warts- A highly contagious virus	Apply a drop of full strength GSE directly on the wart. Then cover the wart with a Band-Aid to keep the wart moist. Re-apply twice a day and continue to do so for a few weeks
Wounds	Mix a teaspoon of GSE in 4 ounces of cooled, boiled water (or distilled water) in a clean spray bottle. Spray wound generously several times a day. You should use a more dilute solution for deeper wounds Be sure to see a doctor for severe wounds.

GSE Baby Care Uses

Used to clean:

Baby bottles

Bedding

Cribs

Clothing

Diapers

Nipples

Pacifiers

Plastic mattresses

Toys

Because a baby's immune system is so fragile it is important to keep baby and everything that they come into contact with, very clean. Grapefruit seed extract is an important tool for killing bacteria, germs and viruses.

Lab tests have discovered GSE to be at least 10 times more effective than Clorox Bleach, Colloidal Silver and Iodine.

The wonderful thing about GSE is how powerful it is and yet it is non-toxic so it can be used safely by babies, the elderly and even people with compromised immune systems.

Many hospitals are now using GSE because of how effective it is and yet it is non-toxic and safe enough for pretty much everyone. It is a safe alternative to the harmful chemical cleaners that have been used for years.

Grapefruit seed extract can be used for laundry to be sure that bedding, clothing and towels are bacteria and fungal free. GSE also eliminates molds and odors.

Hospitals, and even laundry operations that service hospitals, have found GSE to offer complete protection from bacterial and fungal infections that have been linked to linens. They have also found that even after many hours of exposure to the bacteria that are consistently found in hospitals, the linens washed with GSE have been tested and found to be free of detrimental and pathogenic organisms.

Matter-of-fact, hospitals are now adding 10-15 drops of GSE to each gallon of water in their carpet cleaners because it is effective against so many pathogenic organisms.

I wish that this information had been known when I was in the hospital for over 6 weeks. I had trouble with the gowns making me itch because of what they were using on them in the laundry.

It ended up that my mother had to bring me a few gowns and then she would take them home to wash them.

Make sure to *always* dilute grapefruit seed extract

Never get it the eyes- if you do then be sure to flush them out with warm water and contact a doctor.

GSE Baby Health Uses

Cradle cap

Cradle cap is baby dandruff. To treat it with GSE you simply need to mix 1-2 drops of GSE in 2-4 ounces of olive oil. Rub this solution onto the skin one to two times a day until the condition clears   up.

Thrush

Thrush is a whitish coating in the mouth that is caused by a yeast fungus.

To treat thrush in babies you will need to *thoroughly* mix just 2 drops of GSE in 1 cup of lukewarm water. Moisten a piece of gauze with this solution. Gently rub the moistened gauze around the baby's mouth. If it seems to bother baby too much, or you don't have gauze on hand, you can use your finger.

If you use your finger you must be sure to thoroughly wash your hands both before and after treatment to be sure not to spread the fungus.

Be sure to let this treatment sit for 15-30 minutes before giving baby anything to eat or drink,

If baby seems to really dislike the taste of this solution you can put in a drop of peppermint extract to improve the taste.

Kids that are at least 6 years old should be able to swish with the mixture around in their mouth or possibly gargle with it. The nice thing with using the GSE is that if they accidentally swallow the diluted solution it won't hurt them.

The thrush yeast fungus can be found on baby bottles and pacifiers which can cause a seemingly endless cycle of re-infecting if it is not stopped. So, it is very important to treat all bottles and pacifiers with a solution of 2 cups of water add 7 drops of GSE and then soak bottles & pacifiers in the solution for 20-30 minutes and then rinse.

If you are breastfeeding your baby and they get thrush it would be a good idea to mix a solution of 4 drops of GSE to a cup of water. Mix it thoroughly and keep in a squeeze or spray bottle. Use this on your nipples after baby nurses. By the time baby goes to nurse again the solution will have killed the fungus and will be air dried so that the taste should not bother baby. If it does seem to bother baby then simply use a washcloth with warm water to wash nipples before nursing.

It is important to kill the thrush virus at every possible contamination point so that it does not keep re-infecting baby.

Toy wash

Any toy that baby puts in their mouth frequently will need to be thoroughly disinfected on a regular basis, especially whenever baby is sick. This is a good idea whenever baby has had a cold, thrush, etc.

Mix up a solution of 6-10 drops of GSE in a sink full of water and then leave the baby toys in this solution for 15-20 minutes and then allow them to air dry.

Clothing & diaper Wash

It is a good idea to add anywhere from 10-20 drops of GSE (or more) to the final rinse cycle when you wash baby clothing as plain hot water just doesn't kill all of the bacteria, fungus and viruses.

Baby Care	
Bottle & pacifier sterilizer	In 2 cups of water add 7 drops of GSE and then soak bottles & pacifiers in the solution for 20-30 minutes and then rinse
Clothing & diaper wash	Add anywhere from 10-20 drops of GSE (or more) to the final rinse cycle as plain hot water doesn't always kill all the bacteria, fungus and viruses
Diaper rash treatment	Mix 1-3 drops of GSE in 4 ounces of olive oil or vegetable oil and gently rub it onto the affected area
Thrush	*Thoroughly* mix just 2 drops of GSE in 1 cup of lukewarm water. Swab baby's mouth with this solution. Wait 15-30 minutes to feed
Toy sterilizer	6-10 drops of GSE in a sink full of water. Submerge toys for 15-20 minutes. Air dry.

Non-Toxic GSE Household Cleaner

GSE is an all natural cleaning product that has been used to kill common

Bacteria, fungus, viruses and parasites such as:

Aspergillus fungus
E-coli
Salmonella
Staphylococci
Strep
& more

Simply fill a clean spray bottle with water and then add 3-7 drops of GSE and shale well before each use.

To use you just spray the area let sit a couple of minutes and then wipe off or just air dry. You don't need to rinse the area off like you have to with most cleaning products.

Many household cleaners contain hazardous chemicals that your body absorbs through the skin and through the respiratory system. These toxic chemicals are bad for your health as they could cause cancer and other health issues. So using grapefruit seed extract as a natural, non-toxic alternative is a good idea as it kills harmful germs while being safe for us and our pets.

Some cleaners contain dangerous chemicals that can not only cause cancer but do damage to the nervous system. Substances which cause harmful effects to the nervous system are called neurotoxins. These substances can cause neuro-toxic effects which can include the following symptoms:

Neuro-toxic Effects of Some Chemicals

Behavior changes
Death
Elevated body temperature
Impaired coordination
Increased aggressive behavior
Impaired learning
Seizures
Tremors

GSE is a Safer Alternative Cleaner

GSE is a Safer Alternative for cleaning and whitening:

Carpets	Clothing
Eating utensils	Laundry
Linens	Sinks
Tiles	Toilets
Tubs	Wash dishes

It can even be used as a non-toxic wash, as well as a natural preservative, for:

Berries   Fish
Fruits   Meat
Poultry   Salads
Vegetables

In more recent years we have heard of contamination of fruits and vegetables which have made people pretty sick. By using GSE as a wash on your fruits and vegetables it will remove pesticides while killing harmful bacteria.

This GSE wash will leave your fruits and vegetables clean and ready for your family to enjoy with peace of mind.

This same benefit comes in handy with meat too.

And you can use GSE to clean all surfaces where meats, or their fluids, may have contaminated the area.

Other GSE Household Uses

Air Conditioners & Air Purifiers

The filters in air conditioners and air purifiers can hold germs which can then be thrown into the air whenever these devices are running.

This contamination of the very air that we breathe can then be the reason that we get sick.

It is important that we spray these filters with a solution of GSE on a weekly basis in order to kill airborne:

Mildew   Molds
Viruses   & more

Mix 10 drops of GSE in 2 cups of water and put this solution into a spray bottle. Shake well before each use. Spray filters and then let them air dry before replacing them inside the machine and using them.

An anti-mold additive for Paints, Stains, etc

By adding a few drops for each gallon of clear coating, deck stains, finish coat, paint, primer coat, etc. the GSE will make the paint more resistant to molds and mildew.

This works well in high moisture area such as bathrooms.

Antibacterial Soap

By simply adding a few drops of GSE to your liquid hand soap, shampoos, etc. you can make them antibacterial and yet hey are non-toxic.

This is a much cheaper and safer alternative for your family to use.

Carpet & Rug Cleaner

To clean carpets and rugs you should add 10-15 drops of GSE to each gallon of hot water in the tank of your carpet cleaner.

In recent years hospitals have started adding GSE to each gallon of water in their carpet cleaners because it is so effective against a variety of pathogenic organisms.

Canned Food

More recently I have read about how the tops of canned goods can become contaminated by bugs and mice walking across the tops of them. Because of this it is recommended that you clean the tops of canned goods and canned soda pop before opening them.

Mix 5-10 drops of GSE in 2 cups of water and put this solution into a spray bottle. Shake well before each use. Spray the tops of your canned items before you open them in order to disinfect them. Leave the grapefruit seed extract on the cans for at least 20-30 seconds before rinsing them off.

Cutting Boards

You can safely use grapefruit seed extract as a cutting board cleaner. Just apply several drops to a damp cutting board and then use a damp dishcloth to work the GSE into the boar. Let it set for 30 minutes or more and then rinse.

The GSE will get rid of:

E-coli
Fungi
Salmonella
& other dangerous bacteria, parasites and viruses

Dehumidifier & Humidifiers

Use several drops per gallon of water used in these devices in order to control algae growth and kill germs.

Dish & Utensil cleaner

When washing your dishes it might be a good idea to add several drops of grapefruit seed extract to your sink full of dishes or it could be added to the sink full of rinse water.

This is something that could come in handy whenever someone in the household is sick, you have company over and maybe they seem to be coming down with something, etc.

Your dishes will end up shining clean and sanitized which can really when anyone in the household has a compromised immune system.

Eyeglass & Window Cleaner

Mix 3-5 drops of GSE in 16 ounces of water in a spray bottle and use this solution to clean eyeglasses and windows. The dirtier the job the more GSE you should add so for dirty windows you may want to add the full 5 drops or possibly a couple extra if they haven't been washed in a decade ☺lol

Floor Cleaner

Use 10-15 drops of grapefruit seed extract in a gallon of warm water to wash floors. This is especially good when you have young children that play on the floor as it will kill bacteria, fungi, parasites and viruses.

Grease & Tar Remover

Undiluted GSE will actually break down tar and grease as well as other sticky substances. You should pretest a small inconspicuous area first since it can have a bleaching effect when used like this.

Health Care Givers

For anyone that provides health care whether it is for young or old it is important that they not spread germs or take illnesses home to their family.

Because if this it is a good idea to use a drop of two of GSE directly on your wet hands. Rub the grapefruit seed extract all over your hands. There is no need to rinse your hands so you could mix up a solution of 5-10 drops of grapefruit seed extract in 8-16 ounces of water. This could be in a squirt bottle, spray bottle or make your own antibacterial wipes using paper towel in a baggie with thie solution on them.

GSE is so powerful that it is even used to sterilize operating rooms, surgical tools and for the surgical staff to sterilize their hands

Swimming Pools, Hot Tubs & Jacuzzis

If you add GSE to the water used in swimming pools, hot tubs and Jacuzzis it will prevent the growth of algae, bacteria, etc.

Since it isn't broke down by the sun's UV rays, and it doesn't give off harmful fumes, it actually is cheaper and healthier than other chemicals. It is also health promoting rather than harmful to our health

It has been recommended to use 1 ounce of GSE for every 2-300 gallons of water in order to kill any microbes that might get past the ozone.

Water Sanitizer

Whether it is for emergency use or to store water for long term you can use GSE to sanitize the water.

Water should be filtered but if you are unable to do so then at least let any suspended particles settle to the bottom and the carefully preserve the clear water. Add several drops of GSE to each gallon of water. Shake well. Let set for 15-30 minutes and then it is ready for immediate use.

For long term storage you may want to add 5-10 drops per gallon.

Fruit, Meat & Vegetable Cleaner

In more recent years we have heard of contamination of fruits and vegetables. It seems to be becoming an ever increasing problem. There have been a lot of people that have become violently ill due to contaminated foods.

But, by using GSE as a wash on your fruits, vegetables and meats it will remove pesticides, kill harmful bacteria while extending the shelf life.

This GSE wash has been found to increase the shelf life of fruits and vegetables by as much as 3-4 times.

For an easy spray wash like what you find being sold in stores nowadays you can use a solution of diluted grapefruit seed extract.

This will be much cheaper than the store bought stuff and it is quick and easy to mix up.

Food Cleaner Spray

Just add 20-30 drops into a 16 oz spray bottle of water and then shake well. All you need to do is spray this solution on and wait a few seconds. It kills multiple viruses, bacteria, funguses and parasites within 15-30 seconds

Or you can put the solution in a bowl to submerge your fruit, meat or vegetables in and let them set for several minutes. This is the most effective way though it takes a little more effort than just spraying.

For best results rinse when finished. You will be quite surprised at how much filth and dirt GSE removes. Some people have found the water to look almost like milk with all of the garbage that GSE removes from your food.

Produce Wax Remover

This works great on removing that waxy film that you find on apples, cucumbers and other fruits and vegetables nowadays.

Just add 20-30 drops into a 16 oz spray bottle of water and then shake well. All you need to do is spray this solution on and wait a few seconds. It kills multiple viruses, bacteria, funguses and parasites within 15-30 seconds and helps to remove wax.

Alternatively you can dampen your apple, or other food item, then apply a few drops of GSE and work it into the apple till it lathers a bit. Let sit a few minutes and then rinse. This way seems to remove the wax the best.

Miscellaneous Uses	
All purpose cleaner & disinfectant	Add GSE to 16 ounces of water in a spray bottle. This is an all purpose cleaner and disinfectant or antibacterial hand sanitizer. Just spray on, rub all over your hands. No need to rinse it off. Allow 20-30 seconds to kill germs if you *do* rinse.
Regular strength cleaner	Mix 15-20 drops in 2 cups of water. For larger quantity-use 1 teaspoon of GSE for each gallon of water. (Effectively kills E-Coli, Salmonella, Staph, Strep, etc. just spray on.)
Super	For extreme jobs- mix

strength cleaner	30-35 drops of GSE in 2 cups of water. For larger quantities- use 2 teaspoons of. GSE per gallon of water.
Air conditioners & purifiers	Use 30-40 drops in 2 cups of water. Spray your filters every 7-10 days. Let dry before use. Helps reduce the dangers of airborne bacteria, mildew and mold
Cleaner for cutting boards	Use 8-10 drops on your cutting board. Work this in with a wet cloth. Let sit 30 minutes and then rinse. Kills bacteria, E-coli and Salmonella, etc.
Dish & utensil sterilizer	Add 10-15 drops to your dish soap.
Floor cleaner	Use one of the mixes listed

	above, depending in how dirty or whether or not someone is sick.
Humidifier disinfectant	Add 7-10 drops of GSE for each gallon of water. Stops growth of algae & bacteria
Laundry sterilizer	Use 20 or more drops to a small wash load rinse cycle or 40 drops for large rinse cycle for best results.
Liquid antibacterial soap	Mix 7-10 drops of Grapefruit seed extract into 100ml liquid soap- dish, hand or shampoo, etc.
Paint anti-mildew additive	Add 3-10 drops of GSE for each gallon of paint Any more than 10 drops for each gallon could possibly soften the coat of paint slightly). Very effective in high humidity areas & exterior paint

	jobs.
Produce wash	Add 20-30 drops of GSE to sink of cool water. Soak food for a few minutes Or you can add 15-25 drops to 16 ounces of water in a spray bottle. Spray on and let set for 15-30 seconds.
Toothbrush & razor sanitizer	Mix 3-4 drops in a cup of water. Submerge toothbrush for at least 15-20 minutes or just leave in between uses. You should rinse toothbrush before each use. You should make a fresh batch every 3-4 days
Water sanitizer	Add 10-15 drops (up to 30 depending on the quality of the water and how long

	you plan to store it) for each gallon of water. Shake very well and then let stand at least 30 minutes before you use it. In extreme cases you can add up to 10 drops of GSE per cup of water. Can also be taken as a preventative of travelers diarrhea or dysentery by adding 3-5 drops in a cup of water and drink this 2-3 times each day.
Window cleaner	Add 8-10 drops of GSE to 2 cups of water. For larger quantity- mix 40-80 drops for each gallon of water.

Gardening Uses	
Aphid killer Or other soft bugs	Thoroughly mix 20 drops of GSE into 4 cups of tepid water. Soak all plant leaves top and bottom by spraying thoroughly 2 days in a row and then spray again 2 weeks later.
Berry & fruit preserver (extend shelf life)	Spray berries & fruit with a solution of 12-15 drops of GSE in 16 ounces of water. Extends shelf life 3-4 times,
Botrytis Fruit Rot – This is gray mold on Blackberries, Strawberries and raspberries	Mix 1 teaspoon of GSE for every gallon of water. If you need a super strength solution then use 2 teaspoons for each gallon of water. Spray and then wait 2 weeks to spray again. You should spray between the time that they first blossom and the beginning of the second fruit ripening in order to kill this fungus.

Botrytis – This is tomato stem rot	Soak seeds overnight in a solution of 7-9 drops of GSE in a cup of warm water.
Fungicide	Mix a solution of 20-30 drops of GSE into 16 ounces of water. Spray plant & surrounding soil
Houseplants	Spray plants with a solution of 10 drops of GSE for each gallon of water to keep plants healthy & clean.
Hydroponics	Use 8-10 drops of GSE for each gallon of water- to inhibit algae and mold.
Slug control	Mix 20-25 drops of GSE into 4 cups of tepid water
Soil sanitizer	Make a solution of 8-10 drops of GSE for every gallon of water. Use to water seedlings and plants to control algae, fungus & pathogens.
Cut flower preservative	Add 4-5 drops of GSE in a medium size vase of water. Inhibits bacteria so flowers stay fresh longer

Animal Weight - Dosage Chart	
Add the correct dosage for your pets' weight to their food or 4-8 ounces of their drinking water.	
Animals' body weight-pounds	**Recommended Maintenance Dose**
2 to 20 pounds	1 drop of GSE
40 pounds	2 drops of GSE
60 pounds	3 drops of GSE
80 pounds	4 drops of GSE
100 pounds	5 drops of GSE
120 pounds	6 drops of GSE
160 pounds	8 drops of GSE
180 pounds	9 drops of GSE
200 pounds	10 drops of GSE
300 pounds	15 drops of GSE
500 pounds	25 drops of GSE
600 pounds	30 drops of GSE

Animals, Birds, Pets and Livestock		
Internal Uses		
	Antibiotic dose	Give animal the maintenance dose for its size 3-5 times daily.
	Arthritis	Give recommended dose, according to the animal's weight, 3 times a day in

	between meals. If arthritis is of a bacterial origin then you should see improvement within 6-8 weeks. Then give a half dose for another 3-4 weeks. Then keep animal on a maintenance dose
Bacteria	Give animal the maintenance dose for its size 3-5 times daily.
Bad breath odor	Mix 3-4 drops of GSE in 8 ounces of water in a spray bottle. Spray inside of animal's mouth 2-3 times a day
Bladder infection	Use maintenance dose according to the animal's weight. Repeat dose in 3 hours and then keep the animal on the maintenance dose.
Diarrhea	Use maintenance dose according to the animal's weight. Repeat dose in 3 hours and then keep the animal on the maintenance dose.
Fungal disease-mouth	Mix 8-10 drops of GSE into 32 ounces of water. Spray into mouth 3-4 times a day. Use maintenance dose.
Fungi	Give animal the maintenance dose for its size 3-5 times daily.
Incontinence	Use maintenance dose according to the animal's weight. Repeat dose in 3 hours and then keep the animal on the maintenance dose.
Maintenance dose	For a non-sick animal, give the maintenance dose for the animal's size once

	per day.
	See dosage chart for dose requirement for your pet.
Parasites	Give dose daily for 7 days. Wait 14 days and then give the dose daily for another 7 days. Then wait 14 days and repeat again. Then put on a daily preventative dose of half the previous dose
Viruses	Give animal the maintenance dose for its size 3-5 times daily.

Livestock & Pets- External Uses	
Be sure to shake thoroughly before every use	
Algaecide in fish tanks	Mix a solution of 1-2 drops of GSE thoroughly in 16 ounces of water *before* you add it to the tank. Wait 24 hours and then add more if necessary. It is good to keep fish healthy but too much can be dangerous to fish. **Do not add any more than is necessary as**

	it could kill the fish.
Bacterial or fungal skin infection	Mix a solution of 12-15 drops of GSE in 16 ounces of water. *Keep out of animal's eyes*
Birds- sickly All birds- Canaries, Chickens, Parakeets, Turkey's, etc.	Mix a solution of 1 drop of GSE into 4 ounces of water in order to eliminate internal parasites- use this solution for their drinking water. For maintenance just add 1 drop of GSE to 1 cup of their drinking water- be sure to mix thoroughly.
Disinfectant	Use 40-50 drops per gallon of water for cleaning bedding, bowls, cages, etc
Ear infection	Thoroughly mix 1 drop of GSE in 1-2 ounces of water (or you can use vegetable glycerin instead). Use this solution 2 times a day until problem is gone. Then use once a month as maintenance. This is extremely effective for cat's fungal ear infections.
Ear mites	Thoroughly mix 1 drop of GSE in 1-2 ounces of water (or you can use

	coconut oil or vegetable glycerin instead). Use to clean ears. Use this solution 2 times a day until problem is gone. Then use once a month as maintenance. This is extremely effective for cat's fungal ear infections.
Flea & mite (shampoo)	Shampoo fur thoroughly with a mix of 5-10 drops of GSE in a tablespoon of shampoo and then work it into a lather on wet hair. Leave this on for several minutes and the rinse it well. Repeat in 3 days. For really stubborn cases you can add a few drops of GSE to a spoonful of olive oil & rub this solution in to their fur a couple of times a day. Do *not* allow them to lick this concentrated mixture as it could irritate their tongue.
Mange (fungus)	Use flea / mite shampoo mix above, or the concentrated solution, on affected area every few days until the mange improves.

Pet odor	Mix a solution of 3-5 drops of GSE in 32 ounces of water. Use this to spray on animal's fur. Make sure not to get it in their eyes.
Ringworm (fungus)	Mix 1 teaspoon of GSE to 5 Tablespoonfuls of water and spray on the affected area 3-5 times a day. Make sure not to get it in their eyes.
Salmonella	Pets can harbor Salmonella bacteria. So, disinfect their cages, your hands, etc. Thoroughly mix 6-8 drops in 16 ounces of water. Spray with this solution to kill bacteria.
Wounds	Mix 1 teaspoon of GSE to 4 ounces of distilled (or boiled water which has cooled). Spray wounds thoroughly at least 4-6 times a day Deeper wounds require a weaker solution. *Take animal to a veterinarian for severe wounds.*

Important

If GSE gets into the eyes then you need to flush them out immediately with plenty of warm water. Do this for at least 15 minutes. Contact a doctor.

If GSE gets into the animal's eyes then you need to flush them out immediately with plenty of warm water. Do this for at least 15 minutes. Contact a veterinarian.

Sources

Finding information on grapefruit seed extract is not easy. Sure, it is easier than what it was when I first thought about trying GSE but it is still a little known, and undervalued, nutritional supplement.

Over the years I have searched diligently in health books and online to find bits of information about grapefruit seed extract. I cannot go back and find where I got every bit of information as it was meant for my use and I had no idea that I would be writing a book about it. So, I cannot give you every source but I will do my best to list what I am able to.

The Healing Power of Grapefruit Seed by Shalila Sharamon & Bodo J Baginski Lotus & Light Shangri-La

"Extract of Grapefruit-Seed Reduces Acute Pancreatitis Induced by schemia/Reperfusion in Rats; Possible Implication of Tissue Antioxidants". Journal of Physiology and Pharmacology 2004, 55,4,811-821.

There are other publications that we have found that discuss the properties of GSE, they include:

"Alternative Medicine Digest"

"Spraying Chicken Skin with Selected Chemicals to Reduce Attached Salmonella Typhimurium". J Food Prot. 1998 Mar;61(3):272-5.Department of Biological & Agricultural Engineering, University of Arkansas, Fayetteville 72701, USA.

"Articles in "Beyond Nutrition", "Mothering", "Natural Health" and "The Third Option" magazines.

"Coping with Candida", Shirley Trickett

"Parasites – the Enemy Within", Dr Hanna Kroeger;

Antimicrobial activity of grapefruit seed and pulp ethanolic extract. Acta Pharm. 2004 Sep;54(3):243-50.Department of Microbiology, Faculty of Pharmacy and Biochemistry, University of Zagreb, Croatia.

"The Allergy Problem", Vickey Rippere

"Antiatherogenic Properties of Naringenin, a Citrus Flavanoid. Cardiovascular Drug Reviews" Volume 17, No. 2, pp. 160-178. 1999. Neva Press, Branford,
Connecticut.
"The Cure for All Cancers – 100 Case Histories", Dr Hulda Regehr Clark;

"The Effectiveness of Processed Grapefruit-Seed Extract as An Antibacterial Agent: II". Journal of Alternative and Complementary Medicine. Mechanism of Action and In Vitro Toxicity Jun 2002, Vol. 8, No. 3: 333-340

"The Authoritative Guide to Grapefruit Seed Extract", Dr. Sachs

Journal of Alternative and Complementary Medicine 521

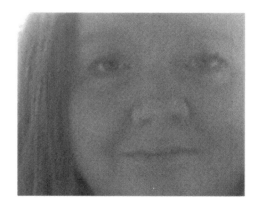

Michelle Oaks has been studying and using medicinal herbs, natural healing methods & remedies for over 30 years. These methods include (but are not limited to) medicinal herbs, vitamins, minerals, extracts, homeopathy, reflexology, subliminal, rife, etc.

Michelle is the mother of a wonderful son. They use medicinal herbs and natural healing methods to stay healthy and to keep their pets & farm animals healthy as well.

You can keep updated on her work here:

http://facebook.com/authormichelleoaks

http://twitter.com/michelleoaks3

This is for each and every one of you...

Dream... Dream BIG and then reach for your dreams. You *can* do it. Even taking baby steps each day is making progress and the more steps that you take the closer you will be to accomplishing your goals.

12801750R00101

Made in the USA
Lexington, KY
25 October 2018